Learning from Our Mistakes

Learning from Our Mistakes

Beyond Dogma in Psychoanalysis
and Psychotherapy

Patrick Casement

Foreword by Nancy McWilliams

THE GUILFORD PRESS
New York   London

First published in the United States of America by
The Guilford Press
A Division of Guilford Publications, Inc.
72 Spring Street, New York, NY 10012
www.guilford.com

Typeset in Times by Keystroke, Jacaranda Lodge, Wolverhampton

Printed in the United States of America

This book is printed on acid-free paper.

Last digit is print number: 9 8 7 6 5 4 3 2 1

Library of Congress Cataloging-in-Publication Data

Casement, Patrick.
   Learning from our mistakes: beyond dogma in psychoanalysis and
   psychotherapy/Patrick Casement; foreword by Nancy McWilliams.
      p. cm.
   Includes bibliographical references and index.
   ISBN 1-57230-817-6
   1. Psychoanalysis. 2. Psychiatric errors. 3. Psychotherapy.
   I. Title.
RC506 .C3196 2002
616.89′17—dc21   2002006982

Note about Distribution: Available exclusively from Guilford in the United States,
Canada, and Mexico. For information about ordering this title in other parts of the
world, contact info@guilford.com.

For Arthur Hugh

When the future is most uncertain it is getting there that wins the day

About the author

Having previously trained with the British Association of Psychotherapists, **Patrick Casement** has been a psychoanalyst and therapist in full-time private practice for many years, and is a training and supervising analyst of the British Psycho-Analytical Society. He is the author of *On Learning from the Patient* (1985) and *Further Learning from the Patient* (1990).

Contents

Foreword by Nancy McWilliams   ix
Acknowledgements   xiii
Introduction   xv

1   Getting there: the unfolding potential of
psychoanalysis   1

2   Mistakes in psychoanalysis, and trying to
avoid them   17

3   The experience of a session: trying to
communicate it   34

4   Towards autonomy: some thoughts on
psychoanalytic supervision   43

5   Some hazards in being helpful in
psychotherapy   58

6   Re-enactment and resolution   71

7   To hold or not to hold a patient's hand:
    further reflections   86

8   Impingement and space: issues of technique   96

9   The unknown beyond the known   110

    Epilogue   126
    Appendix   129
    Bibliography   140
    Name index   145
    Subject index   146

Foreword

Patrick Casement, whose previous writings are now available in twenty languages, has with this book done another good deed for his fellow professionals. Here again, one appreciates Casement's persistent concern with, and increasingly subtle thinking about, issues such as the danger of working from abstract theory rather than clinical experience, the value of *not knowing* despite personal and professional attractions of the wish to 'know,' the intricacies of the process of internal supervision by the therapist, the importance of a non-dogmatic stance in the supervision of other therapists, and the therapeutic superiority of the clinician's wish to learn over consciously well-intentioned temptations to try to give the client a particular kind of reparative experience. Repeatedly, Casement speaks with integrity about the question of authority: its realistic challenges as well as its seductions, illusions and perversions. In this book, he elaborates with his usual thoughtfulness on mistakes: the inevitability of making them, the effort to avoid them and the opportunities they offer to help transform potential disasters into the means of growth in both patient and therapist.

Casement's voice is at once both unique and familiar in a way that recalls Winnicott, Balint and other original thinkers of the British object-relations movement, who can describe the ineffable in ordinary language and thereby bring psychological processes and the psychotherapy experience alive. Like many of the relational writers to whom he has been compared, he is willing to show us what he really does and says in the consulting room rather than hiding his work behind abstractions, generalizations and professional clichés. He has a special talent for putting into words what Bollas might call the 'unthought known' of the psychotherapy situation. In resisting the all too common psychoanalytic tendency to use jargon that creates an impenetrable mystique about therapy, he treats the reader with the same respect that he evidently extends to his patients.

Many of Casement's themes will be familiar to American audiences who have followed the relational movement of the past two decades. Coming from a professional identification with the 'middle group' of the British tradition, he has reached conclusions about authority, authenticity and intersubjectivity that are arrestingly similar to those of American writers such as Aron, Benjamin, Bromberg, Davies, Hoffman, Maroda, Mitchell, Ogden, Pizer, Slavin and Stern. Relational analysts have tended to counterpoise themselves to an American ego-psychological brand of 'classical' analysis, while Casement has respectfully challenged the assumptions of a British version of orthodox technique. Again and again, he argues for a patient-driven rather than a theory-driven version of practice.

All of us who currently make our living trying to be of use to people with mental and emotional suffering cannot help, if we are paying attention and trying to tell the truth, noticing the same kinds of issues arising in our work. Evidently, thoughtful and intellectually serious therapists on both sides of the Atlantic Ocean are finding themselves impressed with similar clinical phenomena. There seems to be a kind of democratization of psychoanalytic therapy, for which Casement is a particularly articulate spokesperson, at work in both England and the United States. In *Learning from the Patient*, Casement extended apologies to authors he had neglected, adding, 'I believe that parallel "discovery" has its own value; and I think that clinical work feels specially validated when a path that others have travelled before is happened upon independently. The difference is that the analyst (or therapist) has sometimes been led to this by unconscious processes in the patient – not by dogma.'

Currently, the dissemination of psychoanalytic ideas has gone so far that no therapist can master even the various traditions in his or her own country, much less those arising in others. In my own case, although I have tried to be a psychoanalytic generalist, I am painfully aware of the pockets of ignorance in my current state of knowledge. For example, I have only a minimal understanding of Lacan, and virtually none of most other representatives of ongoing psychoanalytic scholarship in France. I notice myself envying Otto Fenichel, whose 1945 book could list what he saw as the entire psychoanalytic *oeuvre* of his day. Freud's cherished offspring, the early psychoanalytic movement, has now spawned children, step-children, foster children, grandchildren, great-grandchildren, nieces, nephews, cousins and family friends. Contemporary psychoanalytic writing of high quality is appearing at an exponential rate such that no one can claim to speak for the whole field any more; new theories, paradigms and controversies arise almost daily.

Amid all this burgeoning theory, the struggling clinician is confronted every clinical hour with the challenge of trying to be of help to a particular suffering individual. Above and beyond our personal orientations in the field, we need to describe our clinical experiences to each other again and again, as candidly as possible. As another therapist who has tried to take a 'non-aligned approach,' I particularly appreciate Casement's effort to capture the essence of certain under-discussed clinical processes that transcend ideology. And I think his sobering message about the dangers of dogma is particularly important in the contemporary psychotherapeutic atmosphere, both within the psychoanalytic tradition and outside it.

Within psychoanalytic practice, there is a chronic temptation for intellectually talented therapists to develop new schools, to argue for new areas of superiority, to claim to have transcended and supplanted what has gone before. This tendency is to be expected, given the nature of human needs for recognition and affirmation, and it contributes to richness and progress within theory and therapy. But it also can reinforce our pervasive defensive tendencies to claim an unwarranted certainty, to turn the process of clinical discovery into the process of accumulating evidence in support of our personally favored paradigms and ignoring evidence that contradicts them. I strongly agree with Casement that any time practitioners operate such that their slavish adherence to a particular theory, especially a theory of 'proper' technique, subverts the process of discovery, we are in danger of indoctrinating instead of freeing our clients. Witness the lamentable history of psychoanalytic theory and 'therapy' of people of minority sexual orientation: the damage done to gay, lesbian, bisexual and transgendered patients in the name of psychoanalytic certainty has been incalculable. In fact, as Casement implies, it is arguable that any time we have a specific objective that overrides the effort to understand the patient's personal experience in deeper and deeper ways, we are not really doing psychotherapy.

Outside psychoanalytic practice, there are many other approaches, as there were in Freud's time and before, to trying to help people in shorter, more focused ways than traditional psychoanalytic therapy can promise. The development of biological psychiatry and the cognitive-behavioral movement in psychology have vastly expanded the options available to people trying to relieve their psychological distress. In the United States, and increasingly in other nations, analytically inclined practitioners are feeling relentless pressures – whether from academic critics, government agencies, insurance companies, pharmaceutical corporations, beleaguered mental health institutions or desperate patients – to specify 'treatment plans' complete with behavioral objectives and time lines. Under these circumstances there is a particularly compelling need for practitioners like Casement to remind us of the complex realities of the clinical challenge and the demanding ethical commitments that underlie our therapeutic work. Eloquently, even passionately, he insists on calling our attention to, on the one hand, how little we know, and on the other, how much we can nevertheless help our patients in ways that go far beyond simple relief of symptoms or change in 'maladaptive' behaviors. In doing so, he keeps us both honest and on task.

Nancy McWilliams, PhD
Professor, Graduate School of Applied and
Professional Psychology
Rutgers – The State University of New Jersey

Acknowledgements

I am indebted to Cesare Sacerdoti (previously of Karnac Books) for his insistence that I put together another book; to the many people who have encouraged me to continue writing; to those who stimulated me in the discussion of papers when they were previously presented; and to Nancy McWilliams for writing the Foreword. In addition, I especially wish to express my gratitude to Josephine Klein for her careful editing of the manuscript (as with both earlier books) before it was presented for publication. I also wish to acknowledge the debt I owe to my patients and supervisees, from all of whom I have continued to learn so much, and to express in particular my thanks to those who have given permission for the extended clinical presentations contained in this book.

The author and publishers wish also to acknowledge permissions received to use material that has been published before, the details of which are given in relation to the chapters in question.

And finally, my thanks to my wife Margaret for her tolerance and patience during my writing of yet another book.

Introduction

Psychoanalytic practitioners sometimes slip into a position of arrogance, that of thinking they know best. Thus, when something goes wrong in an analysis, it is often the patient who is held accountable for this, the analyst assuming it to be an expression of the patient's pathology rather than perhaps (at least partly) due to some fault of the analyst's. It is unfortunate that analysts can always defend themselves by claiming special knowledge of the ways of the unconscious. But analysts can become blind to their own mistakes. And even more importantly, they can fail to recognize when it is sometimes the style of their clinical work itself that may have become a problem for the patient.

A major divide has been taking place in psychoanalysis since Freud first demonstrated the possibility of understanding the unconscious mind.

There are many people who are attracted to psychoanalysis, either as a treatment or for training, because the analyst's view of the internal world can be both fascinating and compelling. The analyst and patient can thus enter into a process by which everything can be seen in terms of something else, the analyst being guided by the maps available from theory and the patient entering (like Alice in Wonderland) into this strange new world that is being so richly described by the analyst. The patient may eventually arrive at something that can feel like recovery. But the nature of mental change achieved in this way is sometimes similar to that of conversion, patients giving up one way of seeing themselves for another that is authoritatively transmitted to them by the analyst. A transformed view of the internal world, in this kind of analysis, is sometimes conveyed by a process not so very different from indoctrination, whereby patients take on the mind and thinking of another person in place of their own mind.

My approach to the task of looking into these matters has been to follow, as carefully as I can, my own patients and the work of those I supervise. I have followed clinical experience without looking for proof, or confirmation, of any particular position with regard to theory or technique. I have chosen to be informed by an awareness of the unconscious, together with a recognition of transference and the power of phantasy,[1] and to be guided by a sense that the past is often found to be dynamically present in the patient's current life and in the consulting room. Frequently we arrive where theory might have predicted. Seldom has it been necessary, or profitable, to be guided more directly by theory than by the emerging shapes of unconscious communication.

Approaching my patients in this way, I have been interested to find other analysts telling me of similarities between my clinical work and that of the relational schools in America. I believe these parallels may also be of interest to others, that analysts from quite different beginnings can be led to similar ways of seeing the analytic process, and that this can develop from an independent approach to clinical work just as readily as it can from being informed by a particular school of theory. It is for this reason that I am not citing the interpersonal and interrelational literature, as that was not at any stage what has guided or influenced me during this journey of clinical exploration. In fact, wisely or unwisely, I chose to delay exploring that literature until after finding where this independent journey may have taken me.

This non-aligned approach to analysis has led me to see more of the part played by the analytic relationship in the analytic process, not only as the backdrop to the unfolding transference but also as a powerful factor in its own right. This relationship, as many others have noted, is uniquely a product of the personality of each party: the patient and the analyst working together. It does not necessarily follow universal lines, as might be expected from within a scientific context. It evolves with each patient, with its own dynamic and unconscious purpose. Analysts, if they are not too defended to allow this, can also be subtly drawn into forms of relating that in many ways parallel the relationship between a child of whatever age and a mother, or a child (often older) and a father. Much is to be learned from this, and profound change can result.

At certain stages, as in regression, the analyst may be called upon to be controlled by a patient, as a mother is by her infant. And for an analyst to

---

1 I am keeping to the use of 'phantasy', as used by the British Object Relations theorists to highlight the difference between 'unconscious phantasy', by which we all relate to others in terms of how we unconsciously imagine them to be, as distinct from 'fantasy' which is more a matter of day-dreaming or conscious imaging.

allow this does not have to mean being rendered impotent. At other times the analyst also needs to be firm, prepared to engage with confrontation, like a father with an older child. And the analytic relationship continues in a state of ebb and flow, with the analyst subjected to being pushed and pulled by whatever a patient may be wanting and demanding, or needing, with the analyst (hopefully) remaining sensitive to what the patient may be (unconsciously) seeking to find in this engagement. What is *needed*, however, will not always be confrontation nor will it just be a passive following of the patient by the analyst. It requires the analyst to develop the skills of discernment, to become better able to recognize the kinds of response called for at different times.

In the process of doing what we can with our patients, aiming to hear what they are most deeply needing to communicate, and seeking to understand it, we also try to remain reliable, concerned and appropriately responsive to our patients. In the relationship that results from this, patients may find experience that is new to them. This in itself can be profoundly therapeutic. However, I believe it should never be our aim simply to provide better experience. I do not find that any lasting change results from 'good experience' alone, particularly if a therapist has intentionally tried to provide it. But what can prove to be better, and more deeply therapeutic, is something more interactional than that. This involves both parties in a process that seems to have its own unconscious wisdom and direction, if we learn to tune into it and to follow it. And the clinical journey that ensues can lead us beyond anything that common sense alone could have suggested or that we might consciously have imagined or chosen for a patient (see Chapters 5, 6 and 7).

Through processes of unconscious role responsiveness (Sandler, 1976) and actualization (Sandler, 1993), and sometimes also of enactment (Chused, 1991), analysts can find themselves caught in uncanny parallels with earlier traumatic situations that are being brought by the patient for attention, for working through and for healing. And it can be in the most unlikely ways that we find ourselves getting to where a patient most needs the analysis to reach, if they are ultimately to attain release from what has formerly imprisoned them in their minds.

In this process we will inevitably find ourselves making mistakes, some of which can be quite serious. But in this stumbling we may at times be surprised to discover what we have then stumbled upon, in how a patient comes to use this in terms of his/her history. A continuing theme of this book is therefore to do with mistakes: how to avoid these as best we can, how to become better aware of those times when we are getting something wrong, and how to work with what a patient makes of this.

In Chapter 1 I explore the paradox that psychoanalysis has the potential to free the mind but also to bind it. The experience that may appeal to some students is a dogmatic style of analysis providing a very definite model of how to analyse, which can lead them later to treat patients in a similar way to how they have been treated in their own analysis. But, for patients who have no interest in becoming analysts or therapists, a quite different treatment experience may be necessary and more appropriate.

In supervision there can also be the contrasting models referred to above: one that is dogmatic, spelling out to a student exactly what a supervisor expects, and another that seeks to enable supervisees to develop more nearly their own ways of working with patients. This second model needs to be just as disciplined, whilst still allowing the student a freedom to find ways of working that make sense to them and to the patients they are working with.

In Chapter 2 I offer contrasting examples of mistakes, suggesting ways by which we might become better able to avoid them. I also consider some of the ways in which analysts and therapists can become drawn into making mistakes that become part of the analytic process. This is a theme I continue in Chapters 5 and 6.

In Chapter 3 I offer a single session from an analysis, as an example of my own work in progress. This session has therefore not been selected for any other purpose, as for illustrating a particular theory or a technical issue for instance. It is offered simply for its own sake, being an example of how I try to use the process of *internal supervision* as part of my own working with a patient.

In Chapter 4 I offer examples that aim to encourage students to develop their own process of *internal supervision*,[2] whereby they can learn to monitor their clinical work from the viewpoint of the patient. It is hoped that this will lead to greater awareness of our unconscious tilting of the patient's responses to us, in ways that affect the analytic process, possibly *towards* something that comes from the analyst, or therapist, and *away from* the inner direction of the patient.

In Chapter 5 I explore some of the problems that arise from trying to be helpful in analysis or therapy. I give clinical material to illustrate how a patient can use the analyst's mistakes to reach more of what is

---

2 I originally thought in terms of an *internal supervisor* (Casement, 1985, 1991), but I now prefer to think of this more in terms of a process of *internal supervision*, as an internal dialogue by which analysts and therapists can monitor, moment by moment, what is happening in a session and the various options open to them, the various ways they might respond to this and the implications for the patient in each.

unconsciously searched for. And in Chapter 6 I give an example of unconscious re-enactments (by the analyst), a series of 'happenings' strangely parallel to this patient's childhood trauma. As a result of this repeating pattern of mistakes, the patient was able to give expression to feelings that had formerly been thought of as too much for anyone, as originally (it seemed) with the mother.

The theme of using the analyst to represent key moments of trauma is continued in Chapter 7, in which I explore further the clinical sequence in which I had chosen not to hold a patient's hand. (The original paper being discussed is reprinted in the Appendix at the end of the volume.) More of the background is given here than in the original paper, along with some of what flowed from that central episode in this patient's analysis.

In Chapter 8 I suggest that two technical issues can be of particular help in guiding us in our thinking and our work with patients – those of *space* and of *impingement*. I suggest that if we are to keep the analytic process free from influence, as far as is possible, and from extraneous interruption by the analyst, our being aware of these issues can be especially useful in monitoring how we are working with our patients.

In Chapter 9 I try to convey an attitude of openness, even reverence, towards the unknown that we can encounter in any analysis and which I believe we are better able to engage with when we are not encumbered with too much theory or preconception.

The issue of confidentiality

As always, I remain concerned with the question of confidentiality and the ethical issues that can arise from the use of clinical material from patients' analysis or therapy, and from students in supervision. I have discussed these matters quite fully elsewhere (Casement, 1985: Appendix II; 1991: Appendix II), and I continue to stand by the position outlined there.

I have also been anxious to protect my ongoing clinical work from the intrusion that can flow from knowing that some of this could, even at a later date, be used for publication. So, for ten years after my last book, I remained determined not to publish any further clinical papers. This gave me, and my patients, the true privacy that was clinically necessary. It has only been as I approach my retirement, and am now taking on no new patients, that I have eventually decided to publish some examples of my work from that time.

I trust that those patients and students, whose work with me I have drawn upon, will appreciate the care with which I have sought to protect their anonymity, that others too may benefit from those occasions when

I have had the chance to learn so much from each of them. As before, I trust that anyone who recognizes themselves or their supervised work, amongst the vignettes presented here, will still feel able to choose not to have themselves identified by anyone else.

Chapter I

Getting there:
the unfolding potential
of psychoanalysis[1]

Where are we getting to in psychoanalysis? And how well does the analytic training prepare analysts and therapists for patients who come solely for treatment and have no interest in training?[2]

Introduction

My thesis is that the potential of psychoanalysis is paradoxical. It can either free the mind or bind it. It can liberate creativity and spontaneity, but it can also foster compliance (particularly within a psychoanalytic training). I therefore believe that we have to be increasingly mindful of the ways in which current analytic practice can develop into a false extension of psychoanalysis, whilst to its practitioners it might seem that this has been a true and apparently therapeutic development. But I may need to clarify here that my judgement on what I regard as true analysis is in terms of that which is most genuinely true for the patient, and which is not imposed upon the patient by the analyst.

Psychoanalysis can certainly help to free patients from their symptoms (or some of them); it can help to release them from emotional blocks that have prevented fuller development, so that they can move on from what has held them back; it can help to heal wounds caused by trauma and other bad experience; it can help to bring alive those who have been amongst the walking dead; it can enable the emotionally frozen to become able to

---

1 This chapter is based upon a paper that was initially written for and presented to the Seventh Conference of the National Membership Committee on Psychoanalysis in Clinical Social Work, 'New Inclusions and Innovations', January 2000, published in *Psychoanalytic Inquiry* 20 (1): 160–184.
2 Except in Chapter 2 these epigraphs are are my own thoughts.

feel again, and to live life more fully. It can do much else too that can be celebrated.

But there is one thing that psychoanalysis appears to do almost best of all: it can turn quite ordinary people into something *extra*-ordinary. It can turn them into psychoanalysts! And here is the problem. For, it does not always follow that psychoanalysis (at least within a training context) necessarily releases people to develop their *own* minds and thinking. Within this growing population of psychoanalytic patients, those who are training to become analysts or therapists, there is instead a pressure (however well intended) towards conformity – in order to preserve the 'purity' of the psychoanalytic discipline and tradition, or to adhere to the norms of some revisionist group of psychoanalysts or psychotherapists.

Amongst those training to become analysts, or therapists, there may be many students who are glad to find a clear model of practice in their training analyst. These students may readily identify with this way of working when they, in turn, come to their own clinical practice: even though that style of clinical work may actually not suit their patients as well as it may have suited them. And I am thinking in particular of those patients who are not working in the field of psychoanalysis or therapy. But, if students have problems with such sureness[3] in their own analysis, how are they to challenge it?

So, we can find paradoxical features in this thing called 'psychoanalysis'. We can still find reminders of the *analytic space*, and the singular potential of that, which Freud began to discover almost by default.[4] But we can also find a reinstatement of pressure techniques which, along with suggestion, Freud had ostensibly come to regard as antithetical to analysis as he came to understand it.

From pressure to space

As we know, Freud started by using various pressure techniques: from hypnotism to that of putting his hand on a patient's forehead, commanding the patient to remember. Later, as an advance on that, he changed this to

---

3 There is a paradox here. Some patients may welcome sureness in their analyst. However, when it comes to being understood as an individual rather than as a stereotypical patient, one of a type, patients can experience pressures to comply with the analyst's assumptions or preconceptions. This then becomes a problem, particularly if the analyst resists being challenged by a patient.

4 Stephen Mitchell writes: 'By inventing psychoanalysis, Freud created not just a treatment, but a kind of experience that had never existed before' (1997: 34).

the technique of lifting away his hand, which had previously been pressing on the patient's forehead: as if to suggest he was lifting away the barriers of repression. Later, again, Freud was prompted by a patient, Frau Emmy von N (Breuer and Freud, 1895), to allow her to speak more freely. And through this, the technique of free association came to be discovered. Interestingly, however, Freud even here built in an element of pressure, stating that a patient must say whatever comes to mind, hence the 'Fundamental Rule'. Of this, Freud said there must be *no* exceptions. He adds the point, ironically:

> It is very remarkable how the whole task [of analysis] becomes impossible if a reservation is allowed at any single place. But we have only to reflect what would happen if the right of asylum existed at any point in a town; how long would it be before all the riff-raff of the town had collected there?
>
> (Freud, 1913: 135–136)

I believe it was with the fundamental rule that Freud built in a version of his former pressure technique, even here, seeming to insist that association must be free. But the patient should never be entirely free not to free associate; that is, without the penalty of interpretation!

It is, I think, an interesting and moot point whether the gains in an analysis are greater with the fundamental rule being regarded as essential or whether this too might impugn the analytic space and thereby keep alive a sense of the patient being in some way forced: that is, forced to comply.

Some harmful residues from our history

If we read Freud's clinical accounts with an open mind we cannot help but see occasions when he was seeking to demonstrate, or wishing to prove, his theories. Then, patients who did not agree with him could always be accused of resistance. And he could seem to justify his continued pressurizing of a patient in the name of the patient's apparent need to overcome that resistance. In the end, the analyst could always be right. Or, at least, Freud could see himself as being right whenever he chose. And this has remained a serious hazard in the practice of analysis. I believe this does not happen so often nowadays, but when it does there should be ways by which a patient can hope to be better heard.

Unfortunately, many analysts (like Freud) seem to regard their own position as protected by the certainty of their own sureness. And that may be further protected by the manifold ways in which they can interpret resistance, thus deflecting away from themselves the possibility of their being wrong.

I believe there are many ways in which we can fall into the trap of being too sure in our (assumed) understanding of others. Let's face it: analysts and therapists become experts in making connections. *We can connect almost anything with anything!* And we can always use theory in support of this, however wild these connections might be. Then, when things don't fit exactly, we can assume the patient is employing whatever forms of defensive thinking best lend themselves to our own way of seeing things. For instance:

- If we wish to see the opposite of what a patient is saying as true we can think in terms of *reversal*.
- If wish to address a problem as 'here' rather than 'over there', we can think of a patient as using *projection* or *displacement*.
- If the issue we wish to focus on is not being spoken of by the patient, we can think of *avoidance*.
- If our patient attacks us for something that makes us feel uncomfortable, particularly if it might touch on some unpalatable truth about ourselves, we can call it *transference* or *projective identification*.
- If there is some connection in time we are seeking to make, but it contradicts the detail of events, we can speak of the *timelessness of the unconscious*.
- And if the patient insists that some connection we are making doesn't fit, we can bring in the notions of *denial* or *splitting*, and so on.

In fact, we can use theory in almost any way we wish. And yet there are bound to be times when we do get things wrong, even seriously wrong. Of course we try not to, and it is much better if we don't misunderstand the patient. But if our style of working is that of being too sure, it can become a real problem for the patient when the analyst is getting it wrong (particularly if the analyst is unwilling or incapable of acknowledging this).

If, however, the analyst is genuinely open to correction, there is a quite different security available to the patient. It does not have to be that brittle security that threatens to collapse in the face of any mistake. Instead, another kind of security can be found that is much more resilient, security that comes from the patient finding that the analyst can be corrected, even by a patient. And, if we think about it, the too certain analyst is also defending a brittle security against whatever might threaten it, whether from the patient or from colleagues who could disagree.

Nevertheless, we still sometimes hear of so-called deep interpretation being spoken of as penetrative. We also hear of a patient's resistance to such deep interpretation as *a resistance to being penetrated*. But, we can also see this resistance as a healthy reluctance to being mentally intruded upon, even 'raped'. So, we need to remain alert to the patient's experience of the analyst, and we need to remember that what we observe in a patient can also be a response engendered by the ways in which we, as analyst, are treating the patient.

Therefore, there are several different perspectives that we need to bear in mind with regard to what we observe in our patients. Frequently, they are responding not only to *what* we say but to *how* we are saying it: in other words, to how we seem to be seeing the patient and how we are relating to them.

It is fortunate, therefore, that the interactive and interpersonal dimensions to the analytic relationship are coming to be much more regularly considered.[5] For, if we were to continue to see our task as only that of analysing, without also keeping a close eye on the relationship implications for the patient of what we say, we could easily overlook this interactive perspective. Then, what may in reality come about in response to the analyst's ways of working can be regarded by the analyst as apparently proving the interpretive stance being taken.

It is particularly at times like these that I have come to value the use of *trial identification with the patient in the session*. This practice, or technique, helps me to re-think from the patient's point of view what I have just said, or have it in mind to say, regarding myself critically and from within the sensitivities of the particular patient. This perspective on the analytic interaction can aid us considerably, in helping us not to fall quite so readily into the pitfalls of analysis. For, without this kind of safeguard, psychoanalysis is always in danger of becoming self-proving. Let me give a brief example:

> A patient telephoned me to ask: 'Is it possible to change your analyst?' Sensing she might be into some problem with an analyst, I checked whether she was currently seeing someone. When she replied that she was, I said I thought it would be improper for me to intervene between her and her analyst. Instead, I thought she should continue to discuss the problem *with her analyst*, not with me. If,

---

5 See, for example, the excellent overview of the relational/interpersonal perspectives by Lewis Aron (1996).

eventually, she decided to leave that analysis, only then might it be appropriate to consider with someone else where she might go next. At least that was my thinking on that occasion.[6]

Some months later this patient came to see me, having left her analyst. She began by saying she regarded me as having been 'very slow to understand'. She had asked me two questions, but I had answered her as if she were only asking me one. What she had really been asking me was whether it was possible to change one's analyst *without having to go to another!* She had since found she could not change her first analyst at all, or so she thought, and she was now looking for another. Could I help her to find someone else?

I then learned that her analyst had apparently spent every Friday session interpreting her separation anxiety, and every Monday seems to have been taken up with the analyst's assumptions that she was needing help to recover from that separation. But what the analyst seemed not to allow for was that this patient had been brought up by a single mother who had become psychotic. The patient had then come to feel that the only relief she could ever find from the atmosphere in her home was when she could get away from it. In the transference this patient had begun to experience her analyst as becoming similarly persecutory and intrusive, just like her mother, and she had begun to long for the weekends as the only time when she might find some relief from this. So, in her mind, Fridays had been when she was nearly within reach of that retreat from the analyst–mother, and Mondays were when she had to brace herself for another week of similar misunderstanding from her analyst. But the analyst seemed not to be able to re-think his assumptions about this; so, eventually, this patient felt she had no choice but to leave that analysis.

I have often thought of this example as a salutary reminder that any one of us can get caught into thinking our own way of working is right, apparently not needing correction from a patient. Likewise we can miss something important if we too readily regard a patient's attempts at

---

6 I subsequently came to believe I should have allowed this patient a consultation, even while she was seeing a colleague, to allow her to express her dissatisfaction with that earlier analysis and to explore possible ways of understanding this. That could either have enabled her to confront her analyst more effectively, in order to continue working with him, or it might have allowed her a freedom to leave him earlier. As it turned out, she remained feeling trapped in that analysis until a sufficient crisis, between her and the analyst, finally prompted her to stop seeing him.

correcting us in terms of some assumed pathology of the patient: for instance, as trying to castrate the analyst, or to render the analyst impotent. But it can happen that, with a particular patient, some change in how we are working may genuinely be appropriate: even essential.

Psychoanalytic technique viewed from within a wider context

Much of what has come to concern me about psychoanalytic technique has developed, in particular, from my comparing some kinds of psychoanalytic technique with Winnicott's observations of infants and children, of any age.

For instance, Winnicott observed that an infant, from the moment of birth, already has a capacity for discriminating between an 'object' that has become meaningful and one that is not yet meaningful, and which is therefore being experienced as an impingement. He also noted the importance of a 'period of hesitation' (Winnicott, 1958: Chapter 4) whereby an infant needs to be allowed time to discover the breast, and to find it in relation to hunger that is being experienced so that the baby becomes ready to feed. If an infant is not allowed that period of hesitation, any subsequent feeding is likely to be compliant and without the same degree of zest and vitality. He also noted that an infant can be sensually seduced, in so far as the mother exploits the sucking response to obtain her goal of inducing her baby to feed.

So, what are the implications here for psychoanalytic technique? Of course it can be said that patients are not infants. And even a patient in regression is not to be equated with an infant at the breast, even though some interpretations can be heard as if that is being assumed by the analyst. But what of the manner in which interpretations are presented? Are they offered or are they given? And if they are given too forcefully, what is the patient's response to that likely to be? Does it lead to a real engagement? Or might it rather induce unhealthy compliance? Or (more appropriately) might it provoke resistance to what is being given, a response that could be a lot more healthy than compliance?

Winnicott recognized similar dynamics also operating at later stages of development, for instance in his observations of an infant relating to the spatula (Winnicott, 1941). It is now well known that an infant's healthy response to a spatula that is being put into its mouth is usually to resist it. However, when the infant is left to discover the spatula as meaningful, it can be reached out for and played with in all manner of ways, all of which belong more to the creativity and playfulness of the infant and not at all to the purposes for which the spatula had been designed.[7]

There are important parallels here between the different uses of the spatula and different styles of analytic work. In one style, the analyst seems to see himself as master of the process of interpretation, putting into the patient's mind statements about the transference that seem to be given with such sureness that the patient has little option but to accept or to resist. In that atmosphere, and the analyst seeming to be so certain, there is little room for playing with an interpretation, turning it around, trying it out in different ways.

Playing with an interpretation is very important if insight is to become something more mutually considered and (sometimes) jointly found to be true. Insight that is dogmatically given usually lacks these essential characteristics of play and is likely, instead, to promote a relationship that is more that of master and pupil, with all the attendant risks of compliance and false-self development that go with that.

To use another image, also borrowed from Winnicott, there needs to be room for a patient to *make something* of an interpretation, changing it in the process if necessary, as the patient makes it his/her own. It was in this area of technique that Winnicott devised the 'squiggle game' (Winnicott, 1965a, 1971a), in which he would draw a shape and invite a child to make something of it, or the child would draw a shape and then Winnicott would make something of it – all of this being in the service of creative play. And Winnicott felt that without a capacity to play, between analyst and patient, there could be none of the creative work that he regarded as central to the analytic endeavour (Winnicott, 1971b: 38).

Of course, the needs of adult patients are different from those of children with parents, or a child with a therapist. But the dynamics can be very similar. Equally, however, there will be times when firmness and confrontation are called for, and the analyst must go to meet the need for that when it arises (Winnicott, 1971b: Chapter 11). But, here as well, a similarity continues to be present between the developmental needs of children with parents and the mental and emotional needs of a patient with

---

7 The spatula that Winnicott is referring to here is a tongue depresser, made out of stainless steel, used by doctors when examining the throat. As a shiny new object, usually not met before by an infant, it can either be experienced as something of potential interest, when left to be discovered by the infant, or as something to be resisted if prematurely inserted into the mouth.

an analyst. When things go well, it is the child/the patient who indicates *what* is needed, and *when*. And even the need for firmness is indicated by a patient, as in testing out to see where the limits lie. But I wish to make very clear that I am speaking here of *needs*, not of *wants*.

So, our listening to patients, and our following of the process, can benefit greatly when we manage to remain sufficiently alert to the cues that patients are frequently giving to us, whereby we can sense these changing needs within that process: such as the need for space or the need for firmness.

I therefore believe we are prompted, most particularly by Winnicott, to consider the ways in which we interpret as well as the content of what we say.[8] And there can be all kinds of different qualities to an interpretation, each of which may be seen by the patient as unconscious communication from the analyst, and about the analyst. And we need to remember that it is not only the analyst who is trying to read the patient: the patient is also acutely trying to read the analyst. We therefore should not be surprised that patients note any available indications, in the ways in which we interpret, as to the kind of person they are with.[9]

Interpretations can have the quality of being any one of the following: they can be critical or blaming, manipulative or directive, intrusive or seductive. They can even be contemptuous of the patient, and much else. It is not surprising, then, if a patient begins to wonder what kind of person the analyst is. After all, who speaks to people in ways such as these? It is often, therefore, through an unconscious or even conscious reading of the *quality* of the analyst's interventions that patients build up a quite informed picture of the person they are with. So the analyst is by no means able to remain the blank screen that Freud used to suggest. Rather, the analyst is seen as someone who is capable of treating the patient in such ways as these.

---

8 I am also indebted here to Robert Langs, who similarly highlights this important dimension to the analytic relationship in many of his writings.

9 Fiscalini, writes of this: 'Both the analyst's and patient's personalities, in their unique interaction, are studied, by both patient and analyst. Transference and countertransference patterns are seen as mutually co-created by both analytic participants, rather than as exclusively endogenous expressions of either's closed intrapsychic world. In other words, countertransference partly shapes, and is revealed, in the patient's transference; and, reciprocally, transference partly shapes, and is revealed, in the analyst's countertransference' (1994: 122).

Some implications for technique

If we bear in mind the fundamental ways in which two people interact in other relationships, we cannot afford to overlook the implications of all this for the analytic relationship also. For instance, it is not enough for an analyst to attribute persecutory anxieties to a patient when the analyst is actually behaving in ways that most people would experience as persecutory. And a lot of interpretation can be persecutory, intrusive, controlling and/or impinging.

There are many such characteristics that can be noticed, in relation to the ways in which some analysts interpret, and how they are with their patients. Even though we may be able to see this more readily in relation to the work of others, I think we are all prone to being like this (at times) with our own patients. We therefore have to be alert to that risk, being careful to monitor our ways of working with the patient *from the patient's point of view*.

It follows that, unless we develop this kind of caution in relation to how we are with our patients, we can induce some states of mind that we might then mistakenly regard as part of the patient's pathology. And we will not be able to interpret this away, as far as the patient is concerned. Of course, we can always interpret this away from our own awareness: a manoeuvre that will not escape the notice of the patient.

We need always to monitor our ways of working for what can promote healthy relating and what may hinder it. For, in no other relationship can it be said that it is healthy to have one person so intruding into the mind of another, and being so impinging of the patient, as some analysts seem to be.

I was specifically reminded of this when a patient came to me for a consultation, seeking referral to an analyst. She had already been to see one analyst but she felt she had been 'violated' (the word she used) in the initial meeting with that analyst. This patient, who came from the Far East, had added: 'That analyst seemed to think she was entitled to walk into my mind, without permission or invitation. And she didn't even remove her shoes.' Of course, we can sense very different cultural norms being alluded to here. But I have also been struck by the powerful metaphor in this image, with regard to the degree of respect that we have, or do not have, for the mind and privacy of the patients we see. I think we may all need to be more sensitive to this than we usually are in our clinical work with patients.

Different approaches to the psychotic areas in a patient

There is a common belief that it is only through 'deep interpretation' that the analyst can reach the psychotic areas of the patient's mind. I would question that, particularly as we can sometimes see that this (so-called) deep interpretation may actually *induce* states of mind in the patient which can then be *regarded* as psychotic. However, it does not mean that what is then observed is necessarily to be taken as evidence of something genuinely psychotic in the patient; or that the analyst has been revealing psychotic 'islands' within the patient that less deep interpretation might have failed to reach.

In my own experience I have found that patients, if allowed sufficient mental freedom and space, do not always continue to conceal their psychotic areas. However, when that mental space is lacking, there may be a much greater tendency to keep hidden what *can* be hidden. If an analyst then interprets in ways which are likely to induce psychotic-seeming responses, I do wonder what the gain in this can be. Instead of patients becoming better able to recognize something of their own psychotic thinking, they may see further evidence for believing they are merely responding to a world that, even in the person of the analyst, is behaving towards them in a persecutory way. Let me give a brief example that I have found instructive:

> Many years ago now, a patient of mine applied to train as a psycho-therapist, with a training organization that required a report from the analyst. At the time I was under no obligation to give a report, so I chose not to and the patient was rejected for the training. He then applied to another training organization that did not require reports from the analyst and he was accepted.
>
> Now, largely because of my insistence that I would not allow any intrusion into the analytic space, or any breach of confidence, this patient arrived at feeling safe enough with me to begin revealing the psychotic areas in his personality, which he had previously kept carefully hidden, fearing he would be penalized by losing my support for his application to train.
>
> For a time, then, I was confronted by quite florid psychotic phantasies, which were not induced by my way of working with him but were clearly in contrast to this. Even the patient came to see that. He therefore found himself having to own these deeply secret areas of psychotic functioning as truly a part of himself. And, as

he did so, he also began to discover that I was not alarmed by this, and that what he was now revealing did not change my attitude towards him. As a result, my patient began to find that his deepest secrets could be brought into the analysis and could be safely contained within it; and they could (over time) be worked with and be understood.

Until then, my patient had for some years been working in a setting where he had to take care of psychotic patients. He now began to recognize that he had been defending himself from recognizing his own areas of madness through being closely associated with others, more obviously disturbed than himself, who could seem to carry those aspects of psychosis that he had been denying in himself. By these means, he had been keeping it all in projection. But he now began to realize he no longer needed others to carry the psychotic parts of himself on his behalf. Nor did he need to count upon a further supply of disturbed patients, as a would-be psychotherapist, for the same unconscious purpose of keeping his own madness in projection. He could now face this within himself, rather than having to rely upon seeing madness always in others.

Subsequently, and without any prompting from me, this patient chose to discontinue his psychotherapy training (but continuing his analysis) in order to live a life that was not tied to mental illness in others: all of this because of becoming able to face the psychotic areas in himself, in his analysis. But this had only became possible, I believe, as a result of my providing him with a space that was genuinely free from intrusion from others, and from persecutory attitudes in my way of working with him as his analyst.

So, let us remember that it is not psychotic to feel persecuted when one is being persecuted; or to feel controlled or manipulated, or treated with contempt, when that is how one is being treated. But when analysts are armed with a theory that can deflect their own attention from how they themselves may be contributing to the patient's perceptions of them (as analysts), then serious misperceptions of the patient *by the analyst* are free to operate. And it may happen that the analyst becomes the primary cause of how he/she is being perceived and experienced by the patient. If this is not acknowledged, but is pursued too much in terms of assumed pathology in the patient, then it is very likely to lead to an impasse (Rosenfeld, 1987).

Without adequate self-monitoring, therefore, an analyst can get into behaving like a pathogenic parent, with all the inevitable consequences.

This has been beautifully described by Searles in his paper 'The effort to drive the other person crazy':[10]

> It can be seen that the inexperienced or unconsciously sadistic analyst who makes many premature interpretations is thereby tending to drive the patient psychotic – tending to weaken the patient's ego rather than, in line with his conscious aim, to strengthen that ego by helping the patient gradually to assimilate previously repressed material through more timely interpretations.
>
> (Searles, 1965: 256)

It does sometimes happen that patients are caught in an analysis in which they do not have a sufficient say concerning what is being assumed about them, and they may at times also be exposed to interpretations that cannot effectively be challenged. They then have little choice but to leave that analyst or to capitulate. But if the patient in question is an analyst in training, with the whole training potentially in jeopardy if they leave their analyst, there can be considerable pressures for the patient to come round eventually to seeing things the way the analyst sees them. The resisting stage in this process, if it continues rather than giving way to compliance, can then be attributed (for instance) to some assumed 'paranoid–schizoid' position. And the eventual capitulation (if it occurs) can be ascribed to the attainment of a 'depressive' position. Even though this can fit a particular theory very nicely, it does not have to mean that (in this context) it is necessarily true.

Psychoanalysis and the issue of compliance

In my opinion, one of the most important issues for psychoanalysis, and in particular for psychoanalysts in training, has to do with compliance and conformity. Or, to put it more positively, a fundamental question of analysis is whether it remains genuinely free from pressures on the patient to comply. In this relationship, more than in any other, it should be possible for patients to be free to say whatever is on their minds, without fear of consequence, in order that they become free to discover and to be most truly themselves. At least that is the theory of it.

As already indicated, Winnicott was particularly concerned with the distorting effects upon development, and upon selfhood, which can result

---

10 This paper was first published in 1959 in the *British Journal of Medical Psychology*, 32: 1–18.

from an impinging environment. And it is no accident that those who (like Winnicott) have had most direct experience of the environmental factors in human growth and development, and in pathology, are often those who have most regard for the environmental dimension when they come to work as psychoanalysts. Other analysts, who seem to have been more protected from this direct experience of life outside of their consulting rooms, may have a lot to learn from others who have previously been more immersed in it.

Psychoanalytic training in relation to pressures and compliance

In *Playing and Reality*, Winnicott said: 'Interpretation outside the ripeness of the material is indoctrination and produces compliance.' And, a bit later he writes: 'Interpretation when the patient has no capacity to play is simply not useful' (Winnicott, 1971b: 51).

I have been trying to outline some of the ways in which psychoanalysis has the potential to enable new growth and new life for the patient, and for the analyst too. But, in my opinion, the greatest gains in psychoanalysis are to be found in the arena of the analytic space, within this unique freedom from pressure that can be provided by the analyst. Kernberg reminded us of this in his paper 'Thirty methods to destroy the creativity of psychoanalytic candidates' (Kernberg, 1996). He points out that, if we look at almost any psychoanalytic training, we find all kinds of pressure upon students, not infrequently leading to compliance. How very paradoxical!

Psychoanalytic trainers frequently function as the priesthood of the institute to which they belong. And the priestly function, traditionally, has been to uphold the *status quo* and to keep it pure from whatever may threaten to dilute or undermine it. So, it is not unusual for trainers to teach from a position that can become dogmatic: sometimes with a degree of sureness that can begin to sound like certainty.[11] And we can find this in supervision and in clinical seminars too, as well as in some training analyses. So, how does a student stand if he/she dares to question what is being taught; or, in some cases, how the analysis is being conducted?

---

11 Kirsner, in writing of the move in psychoanalysis towards becoming dogmatic, says: 'The training became the transmission of dogmas and received truths in the seductive illusion of knowledge rather than a method based on ambiguity, unknowing and uncertainty. Orthodoxy was rewarded as psychoanalysts became more devotional' (Kirsner, 2000: 9).

When students in psychoanalytic training are caught in a system of too much sureness, it can become extremely difficult for them to remain true to what is most privately thought or felt. And students sometimes report feeling that if they were to speak out more clearly, particularly if they were to be more critical of the training, they might risk being pathologized by their trainers for not fitting in better with what is expected of them.

A result of this pressure to comply is that some training analyses can bring about false-self change in the student analyst/therapist, and some aspects of training may likewise promote false-self compliance. What can then follow is not only in the area of false-self functioning but sometimes it can also lead to an *identification with the aggressor*. Once such a student is qualified, the next generation of patients may then be treated to a similar stance of certainty, and so the process continues: a process that is then essentially alien to the spirit and centre of psychoanalysis at its best.

So, we come back to some serious questions. Where has psychoanalysis got to in the last hundred years? And are we 'getting there', in the sense of enabling psychoanalysis to fulfil its creative potential?

I believe that, although psychoanalysis does have the potential to provide an opportunity for creative change, and fresh aliveness, it has also continued to develop the non-creative (even non-analytic) practice of using pressure: in particular the pressures of authority. We find this pressuring use of authority in some psychoanalytic practice just as there are pressures prevalent throughout much of psychoanalytic training. But these pressures run counter to psychoanalysis. So, it can happen that, in the way in which we train the next generation of analysts and therapists, we can actually foster some of what is *least* good about psychoanalysis. And some of us may not even recognize that we are caught into this, for we may be passing on ways of treatment that are familiar, and similar to that by which we ourselves had been treated.

Another non-analytic pressure comes from the preconceptions of the analyst, and this too can invade the patient's mental space to the detriment of the analytic experience. The paradox here is that *the more we know, or think we know, the more cautious we need to be in using it*. So, we need to re-find through the patient what we already believe we know. And this more cautious approach to the patient is, in my opinion, much more true to the potential of psychoanalysis than when we think we can take the shortcuts of applying what we now may take for granted, on the basis of accepted theory or of other clinical experience.

Finally, I would like to pass on something told me by a patient. In the course of the work we were doing together, she once said to me:

It is very interesting to find that, in Sanskrit, the word for 'certainty' is the same as the word for 'imprisonment'. And the word for 'non-certainty' is the same as the word for 'freedom'.

We need to remember that, in the work of analysis, certainty can imprison the analyst just as much as it may threaten to imprison the patient. So each of us practising this thing called psychoanalysis is faced with the question: 'Are we freed by our practice of analysis or have we been imprisoned by it?' And the answer, for each of us, may be more apparent to those who know us well than it is likely to be apparent to ourselves.

Chapter 2

Mistakes in psychoanalysis, and trying to avoid them[1]

Anyone who is afraid of ever making mistakes may end up not making anything.[2]

Introductory remarks

One thing that is unavoidable in psychoanalysis is that analysts are often going to 'get it wrong'. Of course, we try not to, but we do need to face up to the fact that we are by no means as unerring as we might wish to imagine ourselves to be. This chapter, therefore, considers various kinds of mistake that are common in psychoanalysis and psychotherapy, and how we might become better able to avoid them. I also want to consider ways in which some mistakes may become an essential part of the analytic process itself.

Little seems to have been written about mistakes made by analysts. However, one of the few papers that does address the subject is that by Judith Chused and David Raphling (1992).[3] Here the authors say:

> An idealization of technical procedures and a belief in perfectibility have kept many analysts from recognizing that technical errors are an intrinsic aspect of the analytic situation. Illustrative vignettes in the literature and case reports used as evidence for theoretical and clinical formulations are written to give an impression of technical

---

1 This chapter is based upon a lecture of this title given in the Introductory Lectures series at the Institute of Psycho-Analysis, London, during the years 1991 to 1994.
2 I heard this many years ago, but the original source remains unknown to me.
3 See also Levenson (1992).

perfection. This fantasy is reinforced by our traditional methods of teaching and supervision, which instill in the student aspirations to flawless technique . . . All this, in spite of the knowledge that technical lapses occur in each and every hour and should be considered an ordinary part of analytic work.

(Chused and Raphling, 1992: 89–90)

Because it is not possible for analysts to avoid making mistakes, it is important that there is always room for a patient to correct the analyst, and for the analyst not only to be able to tolerate being corrected but also to be able to make positive use of these corrective efforts by the patient.[4]

In addition to considering the content of interpretation, and whether this is 'right' or 'wrong', we also need to consider whether the analyst's *style* suits the individual patient, and whether it is too dogmatic or too tentative. And, as already mentioned (Chapter 1), it also makes an essential difference for the patient whether insight is *given* or *offered*. This is all the more important when we remember that personal truth can rarely be understood in terms of black or white.[5] Analytic insight is usually a complicated mixture that may include seeing something from different viewpoints simultaneously. Seldom is it *all* of this and *none* of that; seldom is it *always* or *never*. But that is often how patients see life, so we need to be especially careful not to sound as if we too are thinking of the patient in these 'all or nothing' ways.

We therefore often need to interpret in terms of part-truths, to be explored between patient and analyst, rather than make statements about the patient that can sound as if we see them as timelessly true, or as if we believe them to be true without qualification, such as 'you are . . .' (whatever). And yet we quite often hear examples of analysts who regularly seem to interpret as if they believe they can describe a patient in just such ways as these.

A further consideration about the analyst's style is whether it enables a working alliance; or might it tend to disable this, leaving little or no

4 See also Langs (1978).
5 I often think of the task of trying to understand clinical material, whether in the consulting room or in clinical seminars, as being more like *playing in a sand-pit*, in which we try out different 'shapes', rather than being in a courtroom where the focus is on 'right' and 'wrong'. Of course, there are times when something *is* right or *is* wrong for the patient, at a particular time in an analysis, and we need to reckon with that too.

room for the patient to be working with the analyst/therapist[6] towards some better understanding.

Being dogmatic or tentative

When the analyst works in a way that is dogmatic, it may seem to have the advantage of offering security to the patient who may then feel as if in the hands of an expert who 'knows'. But it can also become persecutory, threatening to trap the patient into a given way of understanding. And that style may needlessly provoke a patient's resistance. So not all resistance that is seen by the analyst is necessarily pathological, to be eliminated by further interpretation. It may sometimes be *healthy resistance* to how the analyst is working, requiring further reflection by the analyst with regard to his/her own contribution to this.

An example

A patient may have been taking up a strong position in an argument with me, and I might have been approaching this in terms of a familiar tendency for the patient to become stubborn, seeing him/her as reluctant to reconsider his/her position. But to pursue this further in these terms might only result in my becoming locked into a state of being at loggerheads with the patient in much the same way as I had believed the patient to have been with me. I might then have to choose between continuing to stand firm, which sometimes is essential, or (maybe) trying to reconsider what is happening from a different position. It could, for instance, be that I have been projecting onto the patient my own failure to reconsider.

So I might say to the patient something like: 'It is not clear which of us is most refusing to shift on this.' The patient could of course exploit my readiness to consider my own part in this, disowning all responsibility into me, which would then need to be carefully examined. Or it might encourage the patient also to step to one side of this potential impasse, just as I am being prepared to do, for us both to reflect on what has been happening between us.

---

6 To avoid needless repetition I shall use either 'analyst' or 'therapist' to refer, most of the time, to 'analyst/therapist'.

Crucial differences also result from whether the analyst is trying to control the analytic process or is following it. The more sure the analyst appears to be, the more difficult it is for the analyst to be corrected by a patient. By contrast, the more tentative style (of 'maybe' and 'perhaps' and 'wondering whether') can more readily engage the patient in a working alliance. But here, too, there is a need for caution about *too often* being tentative, when sometimes a patient does need the analyst to be more firm, even definite. But it does not have to be a straight choice between these two styles of interpreting.

An example

> A patient may fall into being arrogant. If the analyst just says: 'You are arrogant', the patient may well feel attacked by this and may want to argue.

If we practise with this for a moment, trial-identifying with the patient, we can readily see that it would be better if we were to say: 'There are times when you can be quite arrogant.' At least we are then not being timeless in how we are putting this, which leaves room for those other times when the patient is not being arrogant, or is less arrogant than now. This can make it a lot easier for a patient to consider the ebb and flow of this arrogance, and maybe also to begin to recognize the different circumstances under which this *being arrogant* happens, and beyond that to discover the defensive function of arrogance. The result could be much more fruitful then, as part of the analytic process towards a better understanding of the arrogance, than that which is likely to come from the more critical confrontation of 'You are arrogant.'

So, even such a small difference in how the analyst puts an interpretation can make a big difference to a patient, and can go quite a long way towards either fostering the analytic alliance or undermining it. We can usually get a sense of this difference through using trial identification with the patient (in the session), to consider how particular patients might most readily be helped to look at difficult things about themselves.

The analytic work, therefore, is usually better enabled if we are not at the same time provoking a patient into being defensive. That is, unless we have a patient whose character defence is such that we deem it necessary to find a way of shocking the patient into looking at something he/she otherwise might not even begin to recognize.

The point I am making here, in passing, may seem to be a very small point, even a quibble. Nevertheless, I think we can learn a great deal about technique through this trial-identifying with the patient. It can help us to notice those many other occasions when it could be useful to take trouble in adding qualifiers to an interpretation, so that a patient might more readily be able to consider the (part-)truth in what we are saying, without feeling they have to argue with us as if it were never true, because it is not *always* true, etc. But, when I speak of qualified interpretation, I am not meaning we back off from difficult issues. I mean that we can sometimes work more effectively if we approach the more specific from a less focused starting point.

There are, however, times when patients need the analyst to be more sure than tentative, as when there are serious problems in the therapy or analysis. For example, a patient may be indicating that the analyst is failing to understand. When this is the case, the patient needs to hear quite clearly that the analyst can bear to recognize this. Then is not a time to be faint-hearted, defensively saying something like: '*You seem to feel I am not understanding you at the moment*', which can still suggest the analyst believes he/she is understanding but the patient is failing to appreciate this. It may be more appropriate, instead, to say: 'I get the impression I am not understanding you right now.'

This more definite recognition of the problem can at least communicate that the analyst is willing to take seriously the patient's sense of not being understood, whereas a more tentative comment here could seem to be putting the problem back onto the patient, as if it must be the *patient's fault* that he/she feels not understood. And it would be merely confusing the issue to be speaking as if this were more a matter of transference than of some more objective reality between analyst and patient. A consequence, then, might be that the analyst could be experienced as seeming to be unwilling to reconsider his/her understanding of the patient, as if unaware that there could be some actual misunderstanding here. Or the analyst may be seen as being defensive when criticized by the patient. And this view of the analyst often shows up in what follows, in that or in a subsequent session.

Another time when it is important for the analyst to be definite is when the analysis/therapy is in crisis. The patient needs to know this is truly recognized, for only then might there be a chance of adequate attention being given to whatever the problem is, which sometimes will be a problem that has arisen between the patient and the analyst.

Unconscious criticism by the patient

When we are getting something wrong, either in our understanding of the patient or in how we are handling the therapy or analysis, we are frequently given helpful prompts towards recognizing this if we are willing to notice these. It is therefore fortunate that we are not entirely alone in our endeavour to understand our patients. The patient is also present in the consulting room, though some analysts seem to work as if the only source of insight will be found within themselves.

Building on the views expressed by Harold Searles, in his ground-breaking paper 'The patient as therapist to his analyst' (Searles, 1975), and Langs' notion of *unconscious supervision by the patient* (Langs, 1978), I have come to notice how, in so many ways, patients offer the analyst what I have come to call *unconscious criticism*. Basically, I find this occurs in four identifiable forms.

First, and the most familiar maybe, is that of *unconscious criticism by displacement*, whereby we may hear of someone else being criticized, in which we can see that the patient is alluding to something that has been going wrong in the analysis. The following is an example:

> A patient may be talking about an unreliable boss, not knowing where he is with him, experiencing the boss as being inconsistent. We may then notice the context for this, that we are hearing of this after a change of session time, instigated by the therapist; there having been several such changes in the recent past of this therapy.

The second is *unconscious criticism by contrast*. In this, we may hear a patient speaking well of someone else, in particular someone who understands, or who works carefully. It is often valuable to reflect upon this kind of statement, listening for what may be an unconscious prompt from the patient. It could be that we are being reminded that there are others who *do understand*, or who *do work carefully*. We may then wonder about how well are *we* understanding the patient, and how carefully have *we* been working. An example:

> In a session I am feeling confused by what I am hearing from my patient. I am not understanding it. She then tells me about someone at work whom she admires, and says of this colleague: 'He sees the wood for the trees.' This prompts me to wonder what it is that I have not been seeing. It is quite likely that I have been caught up in the 'trees', as it were, while failing to see the overall shape of what my patient has been saying to me (not seeing the 'wood').

I regard this as an example of *unconscious criticism by contrast*. And there are many similar examples that we can each note in our own work with patients, if we keep an eye open for this.

Third is *unconscious criticism by introjective reference.* Here I have come to notice how patients, like children, quite often try to preserve a sense of being well cared for, *especially when they are not,* by taking upon themselves the blame for something that goes wrong. They seem to introject the fault of some other person, then blame themselves for whatever is wrong. The function of this seems to be to protect themselves from seeing that they may not be in quite the safe hands that they need to believe they are in. For example:

> A patient had told me how, when driving, she had a scrape with another car recently, quickly adding that she felt it must have been all her own fault. I then find myself remembering some recent 'scrapes' I have had with this patient and realize that she had been assuming those too to have been all her fault. Perhaps I have been contributing to these in ways I hadn't recognized. This helps me to reconsider these recent interchanges with my patient, and to re-examine my countertransference to her.

I believe we might all find similar examples, from time to time, in our own clinical work if we are prepared to notice them.

Last is *unconscious criticism through mirroring.* Here we may find a patient holding up, as it were, a mirror – pointing to something about the analyst/therapist by unconsciously imitating it. An example from supervision would be:

> The patient (a man) has been getting very upset with the therapist, saying that she doesn't seem to understand. The therapist becomes defensive and, wishing to demonstrate (at least to herself) that she *does* understand, she makes what is meant to be a transference interpretation. She tries to point out that the patient is repeating with her the experience of feeling not understood by his mother. The patient then seems to agree, giving fresh details of how his mother had frequently failed to understand him.

I noticed, in the course of this supervision, that there had been quite a lot of mis-communication earlier in the session. Through trial-identifying with the patient I had already been feeling uncomfortable with some of what the therapist had been saying, sensing that this patient might well feel not understood. Then, with this intervention (given in the name of transference) the therapist has deflected the patient away from something in the session, which could be difficult for *her,* to another time (outside of the session) when things had been difficult with *someone else.*

What I also notice here is that the patient complies with the therapist. He too changes the subject, following the therapist's deflection to the past. I see this as mirroring – *doing what the therapist has just done*. And sometimes this may also (unconsciously) be in the service of protecting the therapist, who may (as in this example) be seen by the patient as having behaved as if she finds it difficult to consider that the criticism might possibly apply to herself, in the immediate present of this session.

In so many ways, we may be able to pick up unconscious prompts from patients. But we will only do so if we are willing to consider the patient's contribution as *capable of being constructive*. If we too readily have a view of the patient as 'tricky', then this positive potential in the patient is more likely to be overlooked. Unfortunately, the patient's contributions to the analytic work are sometimes seen almost exclusively in negative terms rather than positive. I think that essentially critical view can, over time, seriously undermine the patient and the analytic process. And this is particularly true with patients who have come to develop narcissistic defences, which may be in response to earlier narcissistic injury.

An inner dialogue: trying not to get it wrong

As I have tried to illustrate in the previous chapter, I find it useful to sustain an inner dialogue during a session as part of my internal supervision. With practice, it becomes possible to move freely between different ways of considering the interaction between myself and a patient.

I have in mind a model learned from those forms of therapy where there are two therapists, as in family therapy or conjoint marital therapy. When there are co-therapists, who have learned to work well together, it becomes possible for one to risk being drawn into the dynamics of a family, or a couple, even to the point of beginning to get 'lost' in this. At that point, the other therapist may be relied upon to be observing what is happening, to be able to reflect upon this with some understanding and to comment on it. Thus one therapist may come to the rescue of the other.

When we are working on our own it is useful to be able to develop a sense of having (as it were) 'two heads'. With one head we may risk being somewhat drawn into the patient's dynamic. And with the other we can attempt still to monitor what is going on: to reflect upon this, in order to recover a sufficient detachment for us to be able to understand what may be happening, and (eventually) to interpret.

So, within this internal dialogue, I try to keep a part of my mind in a state of trial-identifying with the patient: to consider *from the patient's point of view* either what I have just said or (preferably) what I am thinking of saying. And I find that this can be a constantly enriching experience. For, in matters of technique, we can never attend too much to what we are saying and how we are putting things to a patient.

We can also conceptualize this split awareness in terms of *observing ego* and *participating ego*, similar to that recommended for the patient (Sterba, 1934). Or, we can listen between what we are thinking and what we are feeling. In various ways we can keep our awareness three-dimensional, allowing for lateral thinking as well as linear. This can help us to find meaning that relates more specifically to this particular patient, rather than getting into interpretations that become clichéd and sterile.

Patients will frequently be hearing what we are saying from a different point of view, thus not hearing us as we had intended. I know that we can always try to work with how patients may mishear what we have been saying. But that is not always possible, because patients quite often do not show us directly how they have been hearing (or mishearing) us. And sometimes it is only much later that we discover that a patient has been relating to us in terms of *how* they have (mis)heard us, in ways put together from something we have said that they had not openly responded to.

An example of a patient's response to the therapist's choice of focus

The patient (a female counsellor) has been silent for some time in a session with a male therapist, and she then continues as follows:

PATIENT: I feel that listening to people and counselling them is the only sort of conversation I know. I don't know any other form of conversation other than that; and I am aware of running out of things to say here.

There has been so much to say up to now. But when I am with a man, and I fall silent, the man will often fill the space to avoid being uncomfortable. So I don't know what it will be like here. But I am feeling comfortable . . . well . . . [looking doubtful].

THERAPIST: You have some anxiety about a silence but you also say that you feel comfortable.

In supervision, I note that the patient had spoken of someone[7] who may feel discomfort about silence. The therapist also notes that she looks doubtful when she suggests that she could (nevertheless) be feeling 'comfortable' with him, even though he has remained silent until now.

The therapist tries to acknowledge both the anxiety about silence and the patient (apparently) feeling comfortable. But what about her looking doubtful, which he notices? It is possible she is trying not to give him the discomfort of too much silence with her, so that her continuing to speak might be to make things easier for *him*. Who then is finding this silence difficult? It could be the therapist, who might 'fill the space' to avoid being uncomfortable, just as much as it might be the patient.

The therapist here could be heard as jumping in too quickly, in terms of what the patient *says* about feeling comfortable, as if he might prefer to believe what she says rather than acknowledging the uncertainty in how she looks. Also, he could be heard doing the very thing she has spoken of: *filling the space*. The patient might then read this as confirming her fear that he could be wishing to avoid his own discomfort at this moment.

If I practise with the above vignette I might have chosen instead to wait longer, in order not to be seen as jumping in to fill the space. Alternatively, I might have commented on how the patient seemed to be *looking* when she spoke about feeling comfortable. This might, for instance, have been said to reassure the therapist (the man she is with in the session) suggesting she is not apparently speaking about *him*. So, I might have said something like: 'I hear you say that you are feeling comfortable and yet, in how you are looking just now, I sense that you may not be so sure about that.'

Later in the session I heard the following sequence:

PATIENT: I felt very sad for my father being on his own, so I went to be with him. But he dismissed my support. I didn't mind him crying but he pushed me away. My family were not good when any of us cried. My mother would change the subject.

THERAPIST: Perhaps you wonder if *I* will be dismissive or might change the subject.

---

7 I find that it is often useful to translate what I hear into what I think of as the 'language of someone'. This helps to potentiate my listening, allowing for an easier movement beyond the manifest content of what is being said to what may be latent. And it helps especially in picking up what may relate to the transference.

In the supervision, I commented that I had a sense here of the patient's unconscious supervision. The patient seemed to be saying she was sad that someone (possibly her therapist/father) seemed not to have noticed her support. She may then have experienced her own support of the therapist as being dismissed. Maybe she had seen him as alone in the silence. And, even though she didn't have much else to say, she might have spoken to protect him from feeling uncomfortable with her silence. Perhaps that had been *her support of him*, and I'm not sure the therapist sees that he could actually be dismissing this by not recognizing it.

I also notice that the patient speaks of someone (her mother) who changes the subject when things get difficult: when there are upset feelings around. The last comment here by the therapist could also be experienced by the patient as dismissive, even as a change of subject, from something that could have been more difficult for the therapist to have stayed with: the possibility that *he* could be talking as a way of protecting himself from feeling uncomfortable. It might have been preferable if the therapist had picked up the patient's anxiety about whether he too might be someone who finds her silences difficult, and whether he could also be like her mother in changing the subject.

I offer this example in order to show how we can profitably practise with clinical vignettes, and clinical interchanges, to find other ways of listening to what we hear from a patient and other ways in which a patient might be experiencing the therapist/analyst.

Once again, if a patient experiences a therapist as moving too quickly away from something difficult (for the therapist?) to something easier to talk about, what can follow is that the patient may begin to relate to the therapist as to someone who seems not able to bear staying with the more difficult things that come from the patient. We might then hear of other people who have this difficulty (*displacement*). Or we might hear of the patient as having this difficulty (*introjective reference*). Or we might hear of someone who seems to be able to stay with difficult feelings, perhaps unusual for this patient (*contrast*), rather than deflecting from them as this mother is said to do in the example just given.

Following the patient from more than one point of view

Patients note not only what we have said but also what we have not said, as in our choice to deal with *this* rather than *that*, unconsciously (or even consciously) monitoring what this could indicate of our interest/our priorities/our sensitivities, etc.

This is why I try to follow patients from more than one point of view. And if I too readily think that I 'know' what a patient may be communicating to me, seeing this only in one way, I try to recreate (in my own mind) a sense of *not-knowing*, in order that I can remain open to other possibilities. Then, if I am not able to choose between those different possibilities, this can help me to recognize that I probably need to listen for longer before thinking I am able to interpret.

Quite often I will share my not-knowing with the patient as a way of inviting further joint exploration, or further reflection, on what the patient has been saying, *before* I make any claim to understand it. I don't think anything is gained from a premature claim to know, or anything lost from a continued not-knowing.[8]

A sustained not-knowing is very important too when we find we are working with a patient who begins to feel as if there may have been some sexual abuse in the childhood. It may, for instance, be important to say something like:

> We can't tell, at the moment, whether the indications are that something inappropriate actually happened to you, or whether you are beginning to remember a sexualized *atmosphere* in the family, along with an unclear sense of boundaries.

It is often very important that we keep an open mind around this kind of issue, working carefully with the patient's perceptions. It is, after all, the (internal) psychological truth that we are mainly concerned with rather than objective reality.[9]

Mistakes around boundary issues

Boundary issues are always crucially important. This is especially true in analysis or therapy because the sense of security and safety for the patient depends so much upon the analyst handling these issues sensitively and firmly. And, as Langs has regularly pointed (1978), when there is a problem around some boundary issue it will always be noticeable in the patient's communications – if not directly then indirectly. Langs speaks

8 Of this Winnicott said: 'I think I interpret mainly to let the patient know the limits of my understanding. The principle is that it is the patient and only the patient who has the answers' (Winnicott, 1971b: 87).

9 I have discussed this issue more fully in my paper 'Objective fact and psychological truth: some thoughts on "recovered memory"' (Casement, 1998).

of this as *derivative communication*, meaning the communication that is unconsciously derived from the issue that the patient is primarily concerned with at the time.

There are also other kinds of mistake that can be made in relation to boundary issues. At one extreme there is the mistake of *inappropriate flexibility*, allowing boundaries to be crossed without adequate thought or reflection by the therapist. This almost always leads patients to indicate that they are feeling insecure: not knowing where they are in relation to the therapist, or to the arrangements of the therapy. At the other extreme there can be the mistake of being *too rigid* with regard to boundaries: the analyst or therapist not recognizing when it might be more appropriate to make an exception, rather than working in a way that allows for no exceptions whatever.

We can also notice how patients almost invariably try to make out what may be suggested about *us* by our handling of such issues. For instance, a patient might puzzle about whether a therapist being rigid might indicate that he/she is simply bound by rules, and whether the therapist is afraid to recognize when something more important may be around. Equally, when a therapist is being flexible with regard to technique, does the therapist have problems in being firm or in being reliable?

An example to illustrate the need for adequate firmness

A patient had dreamed that she had been planting her garden with a particular kind of plant, of which she was especially fond. As she wanted me to know exactly the kind of flower her dream referred to, she had dug up one of these plants from her garden to show to me. In fact she wanted to give it to me, so that I could have this in *my* garden.

Internal supervision

As I monitored my countertransference around this, it was not difficult for me to notice that I felt controlled, even intruded upon. And I didn't like the idea of a patient trying to come between my wife and me, claiming a place in the garden which was at least as much my wife's as it is mine. So, this flower could literally come between us, if I were to accept the 'gift' as suggested.

I then recalled what I knew of this patient's childhood: that her father seemed to have allowed an unhealthy degree of intimacy between his daughter and him, so that she had felt as if she had been allowed to be all too successful in her Oedipal wish to claim her father as hers – *thus often coming between her parents*. This sense of Oedipal triumph had left her feeling anxious about her sexuality, that it had seemed to be irresistible, even dangerous. And now she seemed to be flagging this up, between her and me, as an issue to be dealt with, and dealt with firmly. I therefore said:

> I am reminded of how you used to feel that you had been allowed to come between your parents. I therefore believe you may be testing me to see if I might allow the same thing to happen here: for you to be allowed to come between my wife and me, represented by the plant from *your garden* being planted in *mine, or my wife's*.

After the patient had responded to this, pressing me nevertheless to accept her gift, I added:

> I appreciate your wish to give me this present, but I believe it would not be helpful to you if I were to accept it. The plant you have brought to show me really belongs in your own garden.

The patient became very upset. But it later became apparent that she had developed a strongly erotized transference, needing me to provide her with the kind of firmness in handling her Oedipal attachment to me that her father seemed not to have provided in her childhood. Had I accepted her gift I think this could have made it much more difficult to contain her increasing attachment to me. I would have allowed a symbolic repetition of the problem she had with her father. And, in her mind, I believe she would have seen me then as seducing her by allowing her to seduce me, albeit in this quite small way. But, having held this boundary firmly, it remained possible to work through this important phase of her analysis to a better resolution of the problem than she seemed to have achieved with her father.

A contrasting example

> A patient had been unwanted by her mother and was eventually adopted. Later, in her adolescence, her adoptive father had apparently made seductive moves towards her, which resulted in the patient taking flight from the home of these parents. She then began to live in a hostel.
>
> In the course of her analysis with me she wanted to give me a Christmas present: a token gift of a finely carved wooden bookmark.

Internal supervision

I reflected upon the narcissistic injury I might cause to this already fragile patient if I rejected her proposed gift. But I was also aware of my dilemma, as I do not accept gifts during an analysis. In the end I chose to address the dilemma. I said to the patient:

> I appreciate your wish to give me a present. But I am aware of the fact that *presents can create complications during an analysis.*
>
> Equally, I do not want to cause you hurt by refusing this. So, I would prefer to keep the bookmark, which you have wanted to give to me, as *not yet* a present. It can then be something we can think of again, later on, when it may become more appropriate for me to accept it.
>
> When we reach the end of your time here, if this is still something you wish me to keep, we might *then* be able to regard it as a present. But, for now, I will keep it here on the shelf beside my chair – for us to think about again some other time.

A few years later, when we came to the last session of this analysis, I picked up the bookmark from the shelf beside my chair (where it had remained) and said to the patient:

> I will anyhow remember you, even without this bookmark. But, if you still wish me to keep it, I shall of course treasure it as a further reminder of our work together.

She wanted me to keep it, and I could see she was moved by this interchange. I have that bookmark in my consulting room to this day.

Comment

I do not believe we help our patients if we only work to a rule, applying it rigidly rather than with the more careful thought that is due to each particular patient. Patients are very different, so that what may be appropriate for one person could be quite inappropriate for another. But, whichever way we choose to handle exceptions,[10] we always need to follow the consequences and be prepared to learn from them. For we may find important indications in how a patient subsequently relates to us,

---

10 Of course we do need to be extremely careful, in making any exception, that we are not playing into a patient's wish to be treated as exceptional. But not every patient has that problem (see Ladan, 1992).

which could point to a mistake having been made – whether a mistake of rigidity or a mistake of being too flexible.

The most important thing here is not that we should make no mistakes (an impossibility) but that we remain sufficiently thoughtful about the issues in question, both before and after the event. We might have important things to learn, either way.

Some dynamics that can be operating around mistakes

From time to time we fall into making quite striking mistakes. Then, in particular, we need to consider our countertransference to try and find out what our own part in this may have been.

I have found it useful to consider this in two forms: what I have come to call *personal countertransference*, which has to do with our own internal world and sensitivities, and *diagnostic countertransference*, which can give us useful clues about the patient and our responses to the patient (see also Casement, 1985, 1991). There could also be some unconscious *role-responsiveness* (Sandler, 1976) in this, and/or *projective identification* (Klein, 1946), each of which can give us valuable clues to what may be passing between the patient and ourselves.

Often, therefore, mistakes can signal that there is some state of counter-transference which might otherwise have gone unnoticed. The enactment in a mistake can therefore alert us either to something insufficiently processed in the analyst, or to some dynamic emanating from the patient, to which the analyst may be unconsciously responding.

Admitting a mistake

Before ending this chapter I want to consider, briefly, the matter of admitting mistakes.

I have heard it said by some senior analysts that 'the analyst should never admit to a mistake'. Why not? I gather that the point of this is to preserve the attention given to a patient's internal world, focusing on the patient's view of the analyst having made a mistake, rather than the objective reality of that.

However, there is a place for admitting when we have got something wrong. But we have to be mindful of what a patient could make of this, and/or the timing of such an admission. For there is no doubt that we can all too easily be experienced as deflecting a patient's anger if we too quickly get into apologizing. So, once again, we need to monitor the situation from the patient's point of view, seeking the balance that is most likely to be useful to the particular patient. But I do not think it is necessarily useful for a patient to be faced by an analyst who hides behind a relentless silence on the matter of a serious mistake. Neither do I think it useful to find the analyst seeming to behave like others in the patient's experience, who have probably sought to defuse the patient's anger through excessive apology.

We are often going to be getting things wrong. The most important thing, I believe, is that the patient feels free to use such moments, with the analyst being neither defensively reasonable about his/her own mistake nor provocatively unreasonable in behaving as if it had not happened.

Mistakes as part of the analytic process

Winnicott had a specific view on the unconscious dynamics that can operate when the analyst fails the patient in ways that can have an uncanny similarity to the patient's history (Winnicott, 1963b). I shall be returning to this in Chapter 6, but for now I wish to stress that there are times in an analysis when we can get things quite seriously wrong, even in the context of doing our best not to. It is then especially that we can see evidence of the dynamics that Winnicott refers to and which I shall be discussing in Chapters 5, 6 and 7.

With hindsight it might even seem as if we were 'meant' to fail our patients in the specific ways that have occurred in an analysis, because what follows can sometimes become so fruitful. Even though I can't quite support that view, as when the degree of my failure (in Chapter 6) was so extreme as to be beyond comprehension, it is nevertheless extraordinary that we often fail our patients in ways that have an uncanny parallel to key environmental failures in the patient's past history. Winnicott speaks of this in relation to a child patient:

> I must not fail in the child-care and infant-care aspects of the treatment until at a later stage when she will make me fail in ways determined by her past history. What I fear is that by giving myself the experience of a month abroad I may have already failed prematurely and have joined up with the unpredictable variables of her infancy and childhood, so I may have truly made her ill now, as indeed the unpredictable external factors did make her ill in her infancy.
>
> (Winnicott, 1963b: 344)

His caution here serves as a useful reminder that, unless we are very careful, we can also fail our patients in ways that are in *no* sense a part of the analytic process.

Chapter 3

The experience of a session: trying to communicate it

What might we be able to learn from a session that is presented just as it happens, and not selected for any other purpose?

Throughout this book I am advocating the use of internal supervision as an aid to our working with the session in process. Here I have chosen to offer a single session, randomly chosen, in order to provide an example of my own work – including some of the inner dialogue of my internal supervision.

Background to the presentation

Some years ago, the Scientific Committee of the British Psycho-Analytical Society felt that it could be useful if a number of analysts, preferably one from each group,[1] presented a session in close-up detail so that members could get an idea of how each analyst works with a patient. The aim was at least twofold: to have a sense of how an ordinary and unexpurgated session really goes, compared to the carefully selected sessions most usually presented in papers or in the literature; and to have an opportunity to consider the various technical issues raised in such a session. I was one of the presenters in that series.

I have several questions in mind in offering a single session for discussion. For instance, what can we learn from one session about a

---

1 In the British Psycho-Analytical Society there are three groups: the Freudian Group, now known as the Contemporary Freudians; the Kleinian Group, now known as the Contemporary Kleinians, and the Middle Group, now known as the Independent Group (see Rayner, 1991). I am a member of the Independent Group.

patient? I realize that there is going to be a lot missing from any account of a single session. For that reason I give my own passive recall of background detail (as this occurred to me), which I anyhow regard as an essential part of the process of a session. I have noted some of my reflections at the time of the session and I also give my passing thoughts, which are presented here in square brackets.

Also, what can we learn about the technical issues raised by this presentation? I am hoping that this attempt to give a session, in as full detail as I could recall, will allow the reader to consider the technical options (and the implications of these) at various points in the session.

Most sessions that are published, or are presented for discussion, are retrospectively chosen to illustrate something in particular. I am therefore interested to know whether it might be possible to learn something of value even from a session taken at random. What might we find if the analyst is just going about his work rather than preparing for a presentation? And is it possible ever to share such a session – without being influenced by the knowledge of having decided to present it?

I chose a session here simply on the basis of having time immediately after one particular session in which to write it up. But I had not been prepared for what Racker (1957) calls 'indirect countertransference', a response in the analyst that is only indirectly to do with the patient but more directly to do with something else affecting the analyst, such as knowing that he/she is due to present the session to colleagues or for supervision.

At the very beginning of this session, something happened that convinced me that *under no circumstances* could I share this session with my colleagues at a Scientific Meeting. I therefore pushed that idea out of my mind for the rest of the time, deciding that I would find some other session to present. Only afterwards did I realize that I had in fact created for myself exactly the space that I needed. To function properly in the session I had needed a space that was not being interfered with by thoughts of sharing this experience with colleagues. I then became able, after all, to record this *as it had happened*, which is what I present here.

The clinical presentation

A minimum history

The patient was, at the time, an unmarried woman of 29. She is an only child and her parents had both died. Her father died when she was 20 and her mother when she was 25. I shall call the patient Miss C.

Miss C had tried once before to get psychotherapeutic help, around the time of her father's death. She had ended that therapy when the therapist (Dr X) had begun to cross boundaries in the consulting room, the patient then feeling no longer safe in his presence.[2] Miss C had been encouraged by her previous therapist to call him by his first name. I shall therefore let her speak of him here as Mark.

The patient was beginning her second year of five times per week analysis with me. Manifestly, at least, it had been her mother's death that had precipitated a renewed determination to get analytic help.

A Friday session

The patient came into the consulting room and was getting onto the couch as I walked across the room. I had then sensed that she was looking at me as she lay down. This had prompted some recall of the previous session.

The previous day Miss C had expressed a wish to be able to look at me at the start of a session. So far (she told me) she had not been able to look at me at all except when she was leaving. She had emphasized that she was still too afraid to look at me at the beginning of sessions. Therefore, at the beginning of this session, her being *able* to look at me felt like a step of progress.

The patient lay down and started speaking immediately.[3]

PATIENT: Why were you smiling as you came into the room?

[I felt sure that I must have smiled slightly to myself when I realized that she was looking at me. *It was at this point that I felt I could not present a session that started in this way!*]

I did not answer her question. After a short pause she continued:

PATIENT: I feel humiliated.

[I then wondered whether this was because of my smile or because I had not replied to her question.]

She continued:

---

2 It is relevant to say that there is independent evidence to support the patient's statement. Other patients had also left Dr X under similar circumstances.

3 The dialogue of this session is presented here without any significant change. The only changes made are in the history and in the account of my own recall, which have been in the service of preserving anonymity.

PATIENT: I feel that you are laughing at me.

[I recalled that Miss C had told me how her mother regularly used to invalidate her perceptions, particularly if she had said anything that her mother might find difficult to accept as true.]

ANALYST: I think you are assuming that a smile on my face must have meant that I was laughing *at* you.

PATIENT: My mother used to laugh at me, in particular if I was feeling distressed. She would then mock me. (Pause.) She would say that I was being stupid and that I should grow up. I soon learned to hide my crying from her if I possibly could. (Pause.) If you were *not* laughing at me, why were you smiling?

ANALYST: I think you saw my smiling as the same as your mother's, so you experienced me as your mocking mother.

PATIENT: Yes. (Pause.)

[During this pause I had an image in my mind of a child smiling into her mother's face. I was reminded of what Winnicott (1967, and 1971b: 111–118) used to say of the mother's face being 'a child's first mirror'. I also recalled that Miss C's self-image, as seen in her own mother's face, had come to be predominantly negative and self-attacking.]

ANALYST: I think that the problem here is that you have not had much experience of anyone smiling *with* you rather than *at* you.

[I was trying to encourage the patient to reality-test, and to help her to see different possibilities, particularly as the transference to me as the mocking mother was quite paranoid, and I felt this could be difficult to shift. But I realized that I might be experienced as deflecting her.]

PATIENT: My mother never smiled *with* me. She never seemed to enjoy being with me. Instead, she always made me feel that there was something the matter with me, that I was doing something wrong. (Pause.) But yesterday I had just begun to feel safe with you. (Pause.)

Reflection

I noted that I had just been hearing about someone doing something wrong. I also noticed that the safe feeling was referred to as belonging to *yesterday*, not today, so I wondered whether this could be an unconscious prompt for me to realize that we could be on the edge of something that feels unsafe to her *now*. I also wondered whether she might be feeling that I *had* deflected her from the paranoid reaction to my smile. But as I was not yet sure about this I made no comment here.

PATIENT: I expect some catastrophe to follow when I am beginning to feel safe.

Passive recall

I now found myself thinking of her experience with Dr X. I had previously been told that she had begun to feel safe with *him,* and she had been telling him about some of her sexual phantasies relating to him. I had also heard that her father used to ignore her sexuality. But her mother, I was told, had frequently criticized her for any sign of her being sexual, especially if she had ever tried to be at all attractive in how she dressed. She knew that she had wanted Dr X to notice her as a woman, but she had been deeply traumatized when he had begun to indicate some interest in her that threatened to go beyond the professional relationship.

Reflection

Although my mind had gone back to that time with her previous therapist, I did not feel *that* was where the patient was at this moment. The focus in recent sessions had been at a much earlier stage, as she had been very regressed, wrapping herself in the blanket which I have at the end of the couch. Of course, it was possible she might be in retreat from any hint of her sexuality in her relationship with me at the moment. But I did not think it would be appropriate for me to introduce that idea here, as an interpretation, particularly as she has been concerned about whether she is safe with me or not. I also felt she could see a sexual focus for an interpretation here as intrusive, even as seductive. So I chose to be more open-ended in my next comment.

ANALYST: You have repeatedly had the experience of some catastrophe happening to you just when you have had a sense of feeling safe. I think you are fearful now because yesterday you had felt a bit more safe with me than usual.

[What I was referring to was the fact that, in the previous session, she had allowed herself a longer time under the blanket than in any other session.]

The patient nodded and stayed quiet. After several minutes of lying quietly Miss C started speaking again.

PATIENT: Do you like me? (Pause.) You don't need to answer that, and I wouldn't believe you if you said 'Yes'.

[I again wondered whether there might be a reference here to the patient's experience with Dr X, and I noticed the prompt for me not to answer. So I chose to keep my response less focused for the moment.]

ANALYST: Words can be misleading.
PATIENT: Yes. My mother used to say what she thought mothers ought to say to a daughter, particularly if there was someone else present, but I did not feel that she ever really meant what she said. (Long pause.)

[During this pause I wondered whether the patient was seeing me as merely saying what analysts think *they* ought to be saying to patients, but as this would have been a rather stereotyped response I said nothing.]

PATIENT: May I use the blanket? I feel so stupid having to ask each time, but at the moment it still feels necessary to ask.

Passive recall

The background to this was that Miss C had earlier expressed an anxiety about using the blanket, without my permission, as if it might be the same as taking something from me, or taking me for granted. (She could not take such a risk with her mother.) I had interpreted then that she needed to feel that I can give her something with the blanket, in giving my permission, and she had agreed. It had then emerged that she experienced my permission for her to use the blanket as my way of holding her safely. My response to her request for permission had so far continued to be the same as now.

ANALYST: Please do.

The patient unwrapped the blanket and she lay down with this covering all of her except for her head and face. She lay quietly with her face towards me but not looking at me. This was the earliest in a session that she had yet used the blanket. We had about half an hour to go. (Long pause.)

PATIENT: I sometimes worry that you may begin to be afraid of how *very little* I can become here.

[I heard what she was saying in the context of her using the blanket. I therefore felt the reference here might be to the possibility of deeper regression, perhaps even to a level of pre-verbal communication, and whether I could tolerate it and respond to it.]

ANALYST: I believe you are anxious about whether I can accept your need, sometimes, to communicate with me without words.

The patient nodded and remained quiet. I noted that she communicated here non-verbally. After quite a long a pause she continued.

PATIENT: There is something very important about eyes. I feel I can see into people through their eyes, but I also feel they can see into me through mine. I used to feel that I was hiding behind my eyes, afraid to let other people in. (Pause.) There is also something about faces. I need to see the other person's face and (when I feel safe) for my face to be seen.

[I noticed the themes around seeing and being seen, and I was aware of the fact that she had turned her face towards me, but her eyes were looking elsewhere. She is also referring again to *when* she feels safe. As I was not yet sure what to make of this, I stayed silent.] She continued:

PATIENT: Faces were important with Mark (Dr X). I told you about his picture.

Passive recall

She had found a photograph of Dr X which she had wanted to use as a basis for drawing his face. That was before her therapy with him had broken down. She is a talented artist. She continued:

PATIENT: I found a picture of *you* in a journal. I hadn't felt able to tell you about that until now.

[My impression here was that I was hearing about a familiar anxiety, that I might turn out to be like Dr X, also not to be trusted to preserve boundaries. But she was also indicating she was in some way feeling a bit safer with me. I thought I could either take this up in relation to her anxiety about feeling safe (or not) with me as a man, which still might shift the material from her present regressed level, or I could focus on the possible function of the picture which I thought had more to do with her relationship to me as mother. I chose to focus on the latter.]

ANALYST: I think that you are telling me that you have found a way of holding on to something of me between your sessions.
PATIENT: Yes.

[There was a pause during which I could see that she began to relax.]

PATIENT: My mother claimed that *I threw away my own cuddly*. We were on a bridge, going over a river, and I threw it away from me. It went over the bridge and into the river. I never got it back.

[I do not know yet what that cuddly was. It could have been a soft toy but it also *could* have been a blanket, but this is unlikely if it had been thrown into the river. (Even though there had been some earlier references to my blanket in the session I did not want to assume that link.) I felt reminded here of a recurring theme of Miss C being blamed by her mother, and I wondered about her mother's failures to understand those early communications.]

ANALYST: Your mother used to tell you that you had thrown away your own cuddly, so it could be thought of as *your* fault that you lost it. But I can imagine you may have been playing a 'throw away' game with your mother, for her to be fetching it back for you.[4]
PATIENT: I have never thought of that. If I *was* playing 'throw away' with her, she should have realized that and been more careful. She could have held on to it while we were going over the bridge; but she didn't. (Pause.)

[I was again hearing of someone who should have been more careful. I wondered about my own level of care, whether I was being careful enough. But I did not feel there were yet sufficient grounds for me to interpret this in that session.]

---

4 The game of 'Fort . . . Da', which Freud observed his grandchild playing, described in *Beyond the Pleasure Principle* (Freud, 1920).

PATIENT: Do you mind about the picture?

[It was now near the end of the session. I therefore did not think there was time to explore why she expected me to mind. Also, I felt there may have been a link between what she had been saying about her mother (not taking care) and this question. So, I played with the words 'mind' and 'care'. This led to my last interpretation of the session.]

ANALYST: I think you are anxious to know whether I will be mindful of your need to hold onto what links you with me between sessions, or whether I might allow this to be lost, as with your mother.

The patient nodded quietly to herself. She got up and, as she left, she looked straight at me and said: 'Thank you.'

Some discussion

I am not going to get into any extensive discussion of this session as this could open up other issues in this analysis that I don't want to get into here, particularly as I wish to respect the patient's specific permission for me to publish only this single session.

What may be worth pointing out, however, is the value in looking for more than one possible meaning at different points of the session. This often helps us to recognize (as indicated in Chapter 2) when we are needing to hear more before we can have a proper sense of what is likely to be most relevant and true to the patient just then. There are several such moments in this session. Also, there are times when my recall of history (or of earlier sessions) could have led to my deflecting the patient, had I made premature use of that recall.

I hope that I have managed to remain sufficiently aware of how my patient could be affected by my choice of focus, or by what I was leaving out, from what she had been saying to me. I think it was also important that I managed not to assume that her sense of feeling safe 'yesterday' was necessarily still around in the current session; my trial-identifying with the patient also helped me in this.

I won't pretend my internal supervision was always sufficiently alert here, but I believe it was helpfully around during most of this session.

So this is an example of 'work in progress' rather than a session chosen to illustrate something in particular. As such, on this occasion, it illustrates my ongoing attempt at avoiding mistakes in the session. In subsequent chapters (5 and 6) I give examples of when I nevertheless found myself making quite major mistakes, and where I had to work with the ongoing consequences of those failures.

Chapter 4

Towards autonomy: some thoughts on psychoanalytic supervision[1]

How can we best facilitate a supervisory awareness that can most readily become autonomous to the practitioner?

Introduction

We can be helped to learn from our mistakes. And it is in the sphere of supervision in particular that we can learn to develop this process I call *internal supervision*. As already indicated, I find this invaluable in enabling me to follow the analytic process and to monitor my own contributions to this, be they helpful or unhelpful. I therefore wish to consider some ways in which supervisors might foster, in a supervisee, a greater facility in the use of internal supervision as an aid to clinical awareness in the presence of the patient.

As supervisors too can fall into making mistakes, I also mention here some of the things that can go wrong in supervision and how we might be able to prevent this. I shall, therefore, be considering the topic of this chapter from the points of view of the supervisee and of the supervisor.

Paula Heimann[2] used to point out to student psychoanalysts that it is useful to bear in mind, from the very beginning, that one of the aims of

1 An earlier version of this chapter was initially published in *Journal of Clinical Psychoanalysis* (1993), 2 (3): 389–403, and subsequently reprinted in M. H. Rock (ed.), *Psychodynamic Supervision*, (New York), pp. 263–282, and also (in translation) in *Psykisk Hälsa* 2: 114–126 (Swedish) and *Psicoterapia Psicoanalytica* Anno II, Numero 2, Luglio 1995, 12–26 (Italian).
2 The late Paula Heimann was a well known member of the British Psycho-Analytical Society, amongst whose most significant contributions was her seminal paper 'On Counter-Transference' (1950).

an analysis is for the patient to reach the point of not needing the analyst. In many ways the same is true of psychoanalytic supervision.[3]

In my approach to supervision I try to combine three particular aims. I wish to help, where I can, with the supervisee's current work with the patient, building up over time a psychodynamic picture of the patient and the patient's internal world. I also try to give detailed attention to the ebb and flow between the supervisee and patient in the sessions being presented. And I am hoping to develop an approach to clinical work that could be of use to the supervisee beyond this particular session. Thus, I am concerned with both the clinical process and with issues to do with technique. And, even though I may point out times (as a 'teaching point') when I think that some other way could have been better, I always try to indicate why I think so. But throughout I want supervisees to find their own ways of thinking these things through, within subsequent sessions with the patient, rather than to feel obliged to work in any way that might seem to be preferred by me.

The examples I give below are from the supervision of student psychotherapists, but I believe that the principles I shall be illustrating are also relevant to the supervision of analysts and analytical psychotherapists, qualified or not, and so are many of the issues described.

I shall not attempt here an overall view of supervision; but, within the ambit of my chapter title, I plan to focus on a few concepts that I have found useful.

The supervisory triad

The role of supervisor needs to be that of supporting the student *as analyst/therapist to the patient*. This means believing in, and fostering, the potential in the student to become a competent analyst/therapist to the patient. And if the supervisor is not able to believe in that potential then there is already something wrong, either in the selection of the student or of this student's training patient, or in the selection of the *supervisor*.

There are crucial dynamics that can operate in the supervisory triad of the supervisor, the student, and the patient. Overlooking these dynamics can lead to consequences that are sometimes serious and can be unjust.

There are a number of ways in which the supervisory triad can break down. If a supervisor presents too strong a model of how the analysis

---

3 Nevertheless it is prudent for analysts, after qualification, to return for periods of supervision as a way of extending their skills, or at least for occasional consultation.

'should' be done, this can undermine the student's own thinking. It can also foster an exaggerated dependence on the supervisor, so that a student might sometimes feel reduced to being a messenger between the patient and the supervisor, as if the supervisor were the patient's real analyst/ therapist. There is also a problem when students feel that supervisory insights should not be allowed to go to waste, as this can lead to a tendency to use, inappropriately, too much of the supervision in an ensuing session. It is then likely that patients will sense that there is a different hand at the helm in sessions immediately following a student's supervision.[4] The same can happen after a clinical seminar.

When I hear too much of my own thinking turning up in a student's work with a patient, I know that I should not just question the student's lack of independence but that I must also examine my own way of supervising. Am I being too active in the supervision, too directive, too dogmatic? Am I being too critical of the student's way of interpreting? Am I leaving enough room for the student to develop his/her own thinking, in supervision and in the clinical work with the patient? In other words, I need to bear in mind what *my* contribution might be to the difficulties being experienced by the student.

We can see a similar dynamic operating in a training analysis, as both the training analyst and supervisor have a part to play in the triad that supports, or fails to support, the student in clinical work with training cases. Therefore, when I (as training analyst) hear of things going wrong in a trainee's work with patients, I regard this as a prompt for me to review my own analytic work with that trainee. It is possible that some difficulties a trainee is having with a patient may reflect difficulties not being dealt with adequately in the trainee's analysis with me.

When there is something amiss in a trainee's clinical work it is often tempting to question someone else as supervisor, or someone else as analyst, rather than consider our own possible part in a student's difficulties. I therefore think that we should always examine how we ourselves, as trainers, may have contributed to a student's problem before settling into criticism of the student, or of someone else who 'ought' to be helping the student better.

It is also salutary to remember that a mother, especially when feeling insufficiently supported as mother to her baby, can experience her baby's

---

4 It is possible that some patients in treatment with student therapists/analysts could say, if they were to be asked, which session in the week follows most immediately after the weekly supervision.

crying as an attack upon her own capacity as a mother. At times of stress some mothers retaliate. Students can likewise feel threatened by a patient's failure to thrive, being dependent upon the patient for qualification. If at the same time the student is feeling blamed by a supervisor for these difficulties, further inappropriate dynamics can ensue.

Students can have quite problematic feelings about a patient who is raising doubts in the training organization about their eventual qualification. Even though students are careful not to retaliate, at least for the duration of the training, that reaction may surface later (however unconsciously). And one might wonder why it is that some patients end their analysis so soon after a student's training has been completed. Might some of the negative countertransference, which may have been adequately contained during the training, have begun to surface or even to be enacted against a difficult patient once the student has qualified?

Another possible consequence of a student's feeling that his or her qualification is being threatened by a difficult patient is that the student may resort to pacifying the patient in ways aimed to prevent him/her from leaving at a time that would be an embarrassment for the student. This can result in some patients being kept in treatment by means that are manipulative, even seductive, while a student continues to be in training.

Overall, a supervisor, as far as possible, should convey a sense of shared responsibility for difficulties in the analysis of a training case. These difficulties often signal the need for more effective supervisory support, or more work in the training analysis, as much as they may indicate some deficiency in the student. When this dimension of the supervisory triad is overlooked, a student can be left feeling burdened with a problem that can effectively jeopardize qualification.

Internal supervision

There is always a risk that an inexperienced supervisee may invest too much in the authority and assumed wisdom of a supervisor. This can inhibit the autonomous working of a student at the time when it most matters, when the student is with a patient. I have described elsewhere the course of development from external supervisor to internalized supervisor, and the development of a student's own internal supervision as separate from that.[5] It is with this that the present chapter is primarily concerned.

---

5 Casement (1985: Chapter 2; 1991: Chapter 2).

It is not unusual to hear a student in supervision saying: 'At this point in the session I began asking myself what *you* might have said here.' I therefore regard the concept of an *internal supervisor* as representing the student's own thinking as distinct from that of the *internalized* supervisor. Both are important – what the actual supervisor might say and what the student is thinking in the session. I therefore try to foster a supervisee's sense of an inner dialogue between these two positions, so that the thinking represented by the internalized supervisor can be processed, taking into account the immediacy of the present session. Similarly, I consider formal supervision to be something of a dialogue between the internal and external supervisors.

The functions of internal supervision evolve from a student's experience of his/her own analysis, from formal supervision, clinical seminars, and from following the clinical sequence of many sessions. And it is fundamental that students become able to process for themselves what is taking place with a patient, particularly when under pressure in a session, in order to become aware of different options and the implications of each. Interpretation, and sensing when to remain silent, can then more readily become the skill it needs to be, rather than being too much a matter of intuition or (sometimes) paralysis.

For the more immediate processing of internal supervision to become possible, students need to establish a mental 'island' within which to reflect upon a session *at the time* rather than later. This allows greater freedom for a therapist to be drawn into the dynamics of a session whilst still preserving, in the observing ego, sufficient detachment for monitoring the vicissitudes of a session. This capacity to reflect upon what is happening can also help towards making sense of a therapist's affective responses to the patient, and sometimes of being flooded by feelings in a session without being incapacitated by what is being experienced.

Trial identification with the patient

Another technique in supervision is that of encouraging a student to trial-identify with the patient in a session, most specifically to consider from the patient's point of view how the patient might experience what is being said by the analyst or therapist, looking for ways in which the patient's experience might be different from what is being intended. This self-monitoring is essential because it is always more difficult to interpret transference meaningfully if the analyst is also affecting the patient through the way in which interpretations are given: the style and manner, and/or timing of them.

Some preliminary thoughts on the following examples

The examples that follow are intended to illustrate some principles of analytic technique, much of which grows out of learning from one's own mistakes and the mistakes of others.

In these examples I am practising with particular moments in a session.[6] The main purpose of this practising is so that we may become better able to recognize the issues illustrated when we come across these at later times, which surely we will.

Now, a very simple example of a supervisor trial-identifying with the patient can be illustrated in relation to a student's attempts at finding a focus in the transference.

Example

A patient has just been saying: 'I feel that no one understands . . .' The student replied: 'Do you feel that *I* don't understand?'

As supervisor, I took a few minutes to go through this sequence with the student, saying something like the following:

> Let me be the patient for a moment. If I (as patient) have just said that I feel no one understands, 'no one' here could include *you*. I might therefore hear your question as if you have either not heard me properly or as not believing me. So this question 'Do you feel that *I* don't understand?' sounds as if you are expecting the answer 'No'. I (as the patient) could therefore hear this as indicating that you don't like to consider the possibility that I might think of *you* as not understanding. If I feel able to be directly angry with you I might then say something like: 'Don't think you are so clever that you understand everything.' Or, I might feel a need to placate you by agreeing with you, for instance saying something like: 'I am not meaning to suggest that *you* don't understand.'

The student then reported the patient's response:

---

6 I frequently find it useful to think of practising with a clinical vignette, as a musician might practise scales, in order to develop a greater fluency in thinking about clinical issues. There is also value in this for other occasions when, like a musician, we need to have attained a better fluency at the time of actually 'making music'. We cannot take time out in a session to practise, any more than a musician can in a concert.

Of course I am not meaning to include *you*. I know that you do understand really. But my father often made me feel so distant from him
that it was as if I would never be able to get across to him what I was
feeling, even if I shouted. He was always so sure that he was in the
right.

Comment

From a sequence like this it is possible to demonstrate to a supervisee that
the patient's response to this question may well have been to hear the
student as being defensive. The patient attempts to reassure the student,
and follows this by displacing onto some other figure (here the father) a
sense that the student had not been hearing. It therefore looks as if the
patient had been anxious that the student might have to be treated with
caution, as the student seemed unwilling to be seen in a negative light as
(possibly) not understanding. The echo of this problem, now spoken of
in relation to the father, can be seen as an example of *unconscious
supervision by the patient* (Langs, 1978), as if the patient were saying:
'I don't know how to reach you. Will I have to shout before you will
hear?'

An additional thing this student is learning here is how easily a patient
can be deflected from being allowed to develop a negative transference,
thus keeping negative feelings split off from the analysis.

Example

A patient has been speaking of a recent TV programme in which someone
had been telling a psychiatrist that he possessed a dangerous knife and he
was afraid that he might kill someone. The psychiatrist seemed not to have
taken this seriously enough, and this person (in the programme) had then
gone out and *actually* killed someone.

Following this, the patient subjected the student to a persistent enquiry
as to what he would say in court if he (the patient) had really killed
someone. The student proceeded to focus on the question of confidentiality,
saying: 'I think you are anxious about whether it is really safe for you to
be confiding in me, or might I disclose to others some of what you tell
to me?' As supervisor, I felt this was a misleading focus. I therefore made
the following comments:

I feel you are staying with the question of *confidentiality* (and this in
a hypothetical future), which may be easier to think about than the

issue of *potential violence* referred to in the opening statements of this session.

We have been hearing of someone whose thoughts of violence have not been taken seriously enough, phantasy leading to action. If you listen to yourself from the position of the patient here, you might notice that he could be wondering if *his* thoughts of violence are being taken seriously. They do need to be, as the patient is pointing out. If they are not, the sequence might then move into the future with some real act of violence. The matter of confidentiality at such a moment is, I believe, quite secondary to that of how the therapist might respond to the patient's violent feelings and fantasies.

Comment

Again, we can see a therapist deflecting from the more difficult matter that is current in the session. Here it is that of potential violence. The choice of focus could leave the patient feeling that his therapist may also be afraid of this violence. And we need to remember that no patient will feel securely contained when the therapist can be seen as backing off from what most needs to be addressed in the current session.

Example

A male patient has been expressing anxiety about showing his feelings to his female student therapist, particularly in crying. He added: 'It is cissy for a man to cry, isn't it?' And he goes on to say how he has always been very careful not to cry in front of anyone. The student replied: 'You are afraid that I might reject you if you cry in front me.'

I notice that the specific idea of rejection had not been introduced here by the patient but by the therapist. I therefore commented:

> There are two things to draw attention to here: the rhetorical question, which is asked as if it needs no answer, and your actual response. How might you feel, as the patient here, in relation to these two points?
>
> When I listen to you, from the patient's point of view, I could hear your non-response to the rhetorical question as your agreeing that it *is* 'cissy' for a man to cry. I am sure that there is more work to be done in finding out how the patient has come to regard crying in this light, and he will need to discover that it does not have to be that *everyone* regards a man's crying in this way.

Also, where does the notion of your rejecting the patient come from? I do not hear this in the patient's communication. He could therefore misunderstand you as suggesting that, if he were to cry, *you might reject him*. I think it is always important to listen for those ways in which a patient could mishear what we are meaning to say. We can better avoid that misunderstanding if we monitor what we are saying (or are about to say) from the patient's point of view, not jumping ahead of the patient's actual communication.

Comment

I am using this example to remind the student to be careful to notice who introduces what into a session, and that a patient can regard something that is brought in by the therapist as perhaps revealing some unconscious truth about the therapist. This 'reading' of the therapist by the patient can often lead to a patient beginning to relate to the therapist *now seen in this way*, a sequence that is not uncommon.

Example

A patient had been at a school where teachers used to speak of masturbation as 'self-abuse', and he now uses this term as his own way of speaking of it. The therapist reports a session in which she too had been using the patient's own words for masturbation. I commented:

When I listen to you speaking here of 'self-abuse' I am hearing two things that you may not be considering from the patient's point of view. First, I hear you being euphemistic, which suggests that you too may be feeling embarrassed by this. The patient is using euphemism here, as his way of speaking of masturbation, but it will not help him to feel any more able to talk about it if he feels that you too find this difficult.

I am also hearing you as if you too regard masturbation as a bad thing, literally as 'self-abuse'. The point I want to stress is that it is fundamental that the patient needs to find there can be another view of this. It might therefore help to open up the analytic space, in which other views can be considered, if you were to be more direct in your own language – or if you are careful to indicate that you are not regarding masturbation in the same way as the patient. You could then address what he has been saying by referring to masturbation as: 'what you have come to think of as self-abuse'. That could open up some analysis of how the patient has been affected by the attitudes of others in relation to this.

Comment

I am trying to show here that, if there is to be chance of some change in a patient's way of seeing things, there always needs to be a *sufficient difference* between how things are viewed by a therapist/analyst and how they have been viewed before in a patient's life. It is this difference that establishes the analytic space, within which to think about things differently from before. If a therapist appears to share a patient's pathological view on some matter it is likely to seem confusing if the therapist then tries to question the patient's view on this.

Example

The day before the session being reported, a female patient had been kept waiting by her male student therapist. The student had not been immediately available when the patient had rung the doorbell, even though she had arrived on time for the session.

The following day, the patient was speaking about someone at work who had been insisting on her keeping an appointment by being there 'sharp on time'. The student naturally linked this to the previous day by saying: 'I think you are referring to yesterday when I did not open the door to you at two o'clock sharp.' Once again, I felt that there was something worth noticing in the student using the patient's own words back to her. I therefore commented:

> I would like you to be the patient here, to reflect upon how it could feel when I speak to you in terms of being sharp on time. If I say, as you did there, 'I know that I did not open the door to you at two o'clock *sharp*', I think that you might feel rebuked for making a fuss about just a few minutes. At that point in the session this language is coming now from *you*, even though you are quoting from the patient's own words, and it feels like pointing a finger of blame at the patient.
>
> Compare that with the quite different implications if I were to say: 'You are raising the question of punctuality, which reminds me of yesterday when *I failed to be punctual* for your session.' I am unequivocally accepting that it is my responsibility to be punctual, and I had failed in that, never mind the matter of how many minutes

it may have been that I was late. I think that the patient could then feel more clearly entitled to her feelings about my lack of punctuality, rather than being made to feel that she should not be getting upset over just a few minutes.

It may not then be surprising to hear that the patient responded with the comment: 'Well, it was only a few minutes . . . It isn't that important really.' It sounds as if the patient felt that her own view of this failure by the therapist had been treated as not important. She then dismisses this herself, following the lead given by the therapist.

Comment

I want the student to learn here the value of abstracting the more essential theme from the detail. Addressing the issue of punctuality would not so readily lead to a sense of quibbling over how long or short the delay had been.

I also want the student to recognize that there is a matter of importance being presented in the transference, which gets deflected here. The patient is entitled to make a fuss over a let-down of this sort, particularly when it is recalled that she had experienced her previous therapist as unreliable. Is this new therapist about to let her down too? In this session at least, it looks as if that anxiety is being brushed to one side. The patient is thus denied the freedom to explore that negative transference here, which is so crucial to her security in this second therapy.

Example

Another patient had also been in a previous attempt at therapy, with a counsellor, which had failed. One specific factor in that failure was said to have been the counsellor's frequent cancellation of sessions.

Now, in this second therapy, the student therapist has cancelled a session at short notice. The patient has reacted strongly to this and, in the session following that cancellation, she has made multiple references to feeling insecure. She has been saying that she feels her boss wants her to leave; her husband has been rejecting to her; she was late for the session because the bus driver, at the bus station where she has to change buses, had just driven off without giving her time to get on the bus. The student had then said: 'I think that you are, *perhaps*, telling me you are *not feeling very secure* in your therapy with me.' I commented:

I think your patient has been telling you *very clearly* that she is not feeling secure with you. We have heard of someone who may be wanting the patient to leave; someone who is felt to be rejecting of her; and someone who did not want her to be on the bus. Furthermore, this patient has already had to change therapists once. Therefore, the idea that this second therapy could also be in trouble might well make her *extremely* anxious. She might feel in crisis about her therapy with you. She therefore needs to know that you are really in touch with what it could be meaning to her. It might even mean having to change again to yet another therapist.

When I trial-identify with the patient here, your use of 'perhaps' suggests to me that you are not really registering what a crisis this could be for the patient. Also, 'not feeling very secure' sounds as if you are again minimizing the insecurity the patient could be feeling. If you had listened to what you had in mind to say here, from the patient's point of view, you could have picked up these points for yourself.

Comment ·

I make a lot of this small detail as a teaching point. There will certainly be other occasions when this therapist will need to be more firm than tentative, so it is worth learning about this now because a patient who is in crisis needs to have a clear sense of the analyst/therapist being genuinely in touch with this fact, feeling some of the impact of that crisis as well. It is not enough to be commenting, as it were, from afar. But the opposite problem exists too – that of the therapist appearing too sure, as in the following example.

Example

A patient has been describing a row with his wife after which she had walked out. The student therapist said: 'You must have felt very rejected.' The patient replied: 'I suppose so', and continued to talk about feeling that his wife had just not understood what the row had been about. I commented:

I am concerned about two things here. First, you say that the patient 'must have' felt rejected. Why *must* he have felt that? I think you may have put yourself too literally into the patient's shoes here.

When we attempt to trial-identify with the patient, we need always to bear in mind that we are not literally putting *ourselves* into the patient's shoes. That is almost bound to be misleading, as we are then likely to note what *we* might have felt in that situation rather than what *the patient* may have felt. So, in trial-identifying, we need to use all that we know about the patient in trying to explore what the patient (with the patient's particular experience and history) might feel in that situation.

Then, drawing upon my memory of recent sessions with this patient, I continued:

If we bear in mind what else we know about this patient, we may remember that he has been playing with the idea of provoking his wife to leave, with a view to staying in the marital home and bringing his girlfriend in to live there with him. He also likes putting his wife in the wrong. So, he may well have felt all sorts of other things here than just feeling rejected. For instance, he might have felt triumph.

As we actually do not know what this patient felt, we might be able to help him to reflect upon his *own* feelings here. It would have been enough to say: 'It is not clear what you felt about her leaving.' The patient could then begin to clarify this, if he wishes. And, in this particular session, I then hear the patient replying that he felt not understood by someone. That could be some unconscious supervision by the patient. He may have felt not understood by you.

Comment

In my response here I am, as so often, teaching about technique. But, in addition, I find myself using the plural 'we'. I have sometimes thought of this as *the plural of supervision*. I try not to stay too much with 'I' and 'you', as if I am telling the supervisee what he/she might say. I think that can all too easily be experienced as undermining, even persecutory. I am therefore putting myself alongside the supervisee, trying to consider different options, speaking of what 'we' might notice and what 'we' might say.

I am also illustrating here the value of using a stance of not-knowing as a way of encouraging the patient to reflect. We are frequently in a position where we cannot be that certain, so it is necessary to develop ways of enabling the process of joint exploration with the patient. And it does not have to be just a matter of asking questions, which can be experienced as intrusive and controlling.

I also wish to note here that I am not yet addressing the much larger issue of the patient's ruthless treatment of his wife, which clearly needs extensive attention in the therapy. As a step towards that further work, I am concerned here with the student's deflection from that issue through his assuming that he knows what the patient 'must' have felt, and that this must have been to do with being rejected.

Example

A patient has been in therapy for two years as a student training case. The patient is now talking of ending. At one point in a session the student reports having said: 'I think that you are taking flight into health because you are afraid of what else we need to face in your therapy. And, if you take flight from this, you will find that you can't get away from yourself and you will eventually regret ending prematurely.' I commented:

> I am unhappy about this for a number of reasons. First, 'flight into health' is jargon. Could we not find some other way of addressing this so that we do not invite an intellectualization of the problem? Second, we do not *know* why this patient is wanting to leave. It could be that she is anxious about whether she will be less welcome as a low-fee patient when she has served her time as a training case. (She had discovered early in her treatment that her therapist was a student.) Third, you build upon your untested hypothesis (that this is flight into health) before you have determined whether that is even a relevant point here. And then you can be heard as threatening the patient with internal consequences if she leaves.

Comment

I think there are some object lessons to notice here. Some students do slip into intellectualizing the process, with the use of jargon as part of that. Also, I want the student to notice when there is an untested hypothesis already being built on, which can easily turn into a 'two-tier interpretation'. And I want the student to recognize the need to explore what the various strands might be in this idea of leaving now, as there are likely to be several elements in this, not just one. In addition, we need to notice when an interpretation can be experienced as a threat, and not only as a cautionary warning. Patients can be very seriously disturbed by this kind of comment, and the therapist's contribution to that disturbance is, I think, sometimes overlooked.

Concluding remarks

As well as illustrating some specific technical issues, I have been trying to give an idea of a general atmosphere that encourages students to learn about technique for themselves, within the ongoing process of a session.

Another step in this, not illustrated here, is to encourage students to share their own thoughts of internal supervision as an integral part of their presentation of a session.

For analysts and therapists, as well as students, there will always be more to learn about technique. In most sessions there are technical points to notice and different ways of dealing with them. Learning to trial-identify with the patient is therefore a necessary step in learning to recognize what the issues are, the different options and the implications of each for the patient. This can then become a natural part of the process of internal supervision, which can become the heir to formal supervision.

These are some of the ways in which we can foster the autonomy that students need to have begun to acquire before being qualified to work without supervision. There will, of course, be much else that is necessary in any supervision of a student therapist/analyst beyond what has been discussed here, but I am hoping that the points made thus far could be found to be useful.

Chapter 5

Some hazards in being helpful in psychotherapy[1]

It often happens in analysis and psychotherapy that we particularly fail to help when we are most trying to be helpful.

Introduction

The idea of being helpful to others naturally plays a part in attracting people into the helping professions. And some of these people then move on to become psychotherapists. But it can happen that a residue of that early and sometimes quite naive wish to be helpful may remain over-active, to the detriment of what therapists then do *with* and *for* their patients. Along with this, there is a kind of 'twin' wish to be *seen as helpful*, which can also become an obstacle to working firmly enough within the negative transference when that is where the therapeutic work most needs to be.

It is of course understandable that we should try to find ways of helping those who come to us in distress. But it is also a clinical fact that what can turn out to be most helpful to a patient *in the long term* is not necessarily that which the therapist might most readily think of as likely to help.

So, why is this issue so complex?

1 First presented to the Psychotherapy Section and Scientific Meeting of the British Psychological Society on Saturday, 29 January 2000 (at University of Westminster Union, Regent Street, London), when the theme of the day had been 'Being Helpful in Psychotherapy'. An earlier version of this paper was published in The British Psychological Society's *Psychotherapy Section Newsletter*, No. 28, September 2000.

Dealing with an impasse

Not infrequently we hear of a therapist who has used some exceptional manoeuvre to help a patient to get through a crisis or an impasse in the therapy. Often this is because of some unbearable tension or pressure being experienced within the therapeutic relationship. And it is not unusual for therapists then to come up with unorthodox ways of trying to resolve this. For example, the therapist may lay a hand on the patient's arm or shoulder, or may take the patient's hand. Or the therapist may lend the patient some object from the consulting room to take home as a kind of transitional object. Or the therapist offers some exceptional access over a weekend, or during a holiday period.

Examples of such ways of trying to help patients, especially at a time of stress or crisis, are manifold. But one problem then is that none of us is in a position really to assess from afar the dynamics operating in someone else's clinical work, or to assess the ensuing sequence from a distance, as we were not working with the patient in question. Also, it is so very easy to be wise after the event, especially when we are considering a case that is not our own. And there are plenty of examples, which seem convincing in the way they are presented, where some major crisis appears to have been averted through such exceptional ways. So, who are we to criticize?

I am reluctant to find fault with what others have done when trying to deal with a crisis, for they may have saved a patient from something far worse had they not acted as they did. But what I *do* want to consider are the dynamics that can be operating at times like these, so that we may be able to assess such times differently, for ourselves, when we find that we are caught into something similar.

Intended helpfulness

It may be useful to compare the dynamics of *trying to be helpful* with the dynamics of *trying to reassure*.

We often hear it said (in psychoanalytic circles) that 'reassurance never reassures', and I believe that to be true. At least, in my experience, I find that the only person ever likely to *be* reassured by such a manoeuvre is the person who is trying to give the reassurance.

Example

A male therapist wants to help his female patient to get through the summer break in therapy. So, wanting to believe she will get through this break without undue crisis, he says to her: 'I believe you will be all right until I see you after the break.'

Now, if we look at this from the point of view of the patient, it is not difficult to imagine that she could experience this at two quite different levels. Consciously, she might indeed feel reassured that her therapist believes in her capacity to manage without him during the break. But the effect of this might only be superficial. At a deeper level, she could also sense that he wants to be able to go on holiday without having to be worried about her while he is away. He can also be heard as addressing the state of mind *he wants to find* in his patient: not necessarily the state of mind *she is actually in.*

When the patient is anyhow feeling anxious about getting through the holiday break, without access to her therapist, she could feel even more anxious because of hearing that he seems to be wishing to believe she will be all right. The implications of this might feel quite distanced from what she could then be feeling. And if the patient is really to feel helped through the break, she is more likely to feel this if she senses that her therapist remains mindful of what she is *actually* feeling rather than what he may *want* her to feel.

Another problem with this comment is that it speaks to only one level in the patient. But frequently the patient has different feelings at different levels, especially when there has been regression in the therapy. An alternative to reassurance here (which I only found through learning from my own mistakes over this kind of issue) could be to acknowledge more clearly how the patient might be feeling, also taking into account the possibility of there being different levels to this.

Example

I once said to a patient, before a long summer break, 'We both know that, as an adult, you will find ways of coping while I am away. But you may nevertheless feel that, *if I really understood* what my prolonged absence could feel like to the child in you, I would not be *able* to go.'

Comment

This patient, who had never cried before in his analysis, was in tears after I said this. He sensed that maybe I *did* have some idea of what my absence could mean to him, particularly in the light of his childhood experience of absences and abandonment. Any attempt at reassurance here would only have confirmed his suspicion that I was out of touch with what he actually felt in his inner regressed state.

What the patient makes of the therapist's attempts at being helpful

It is always likely that a patient will read a therapist's attempts at being helpful in terms of what this could mean to the therapist, in addition to what it is intended to mean to the patient. Sometimes, it can result in a patient experiencing this in terms quite other than how it had been intended, along the lines already illustrated.

At other times this reading by a patient of the therapist's intention does not matter so much, as in the following vignette.

Example

I once heard a psychoanalyst tell of an occasion when he had been visiting a female patient in hospital where she was being treated for a terminal illness. He had been visiting her daily so that she could continue her analysis without interruption.

On one occasion, the analyst arrived to find that the previous visitor had put some flowers at the end of the bed. As it was a very hot day, the previous visitor having only just left, the analyst offered to find a nurse who could put the visitor's flowers in water – before starting the session. But the patient seemed to react to this with alarm, saying: 'The flowers can wait. A nurse will attend to them later.'

Comment

Reflecting upon the patient's response, one can hear her reacting as if her own need of the session might be in danger of being put second to some need of the flowers. She could be saying: 'The flowers can wait, but what about *me*?' She could also have been pointing out that putting flowers in water was more appropriate for a nurse to do than for her psychoanalyst.

On his way back from the hospital the analyst had reflected upon his patient's alarm. She seemed to have been shocked that he had acted out of role, offering to get the flowers put into water, which was quite out of line with his usual way of being with her. He decided to bring this up during the next session. In the following session, the analyst mentioned that he had noticed the patient's shocked reaction to his offer to find water for the flowers. She replied: 'That is quite all right doctor. I do understand. *I know you don't want me to die.*'

This example shows us a patient reading the mind of the professional who is treating her, recognizing very accurately part of what had motivated him. However, in this illustration, it is unlikely that anything but good came out of this moment of unconscious self-revelation by the analyst. But the reading of the analyst by a patient *at other times* can have a much more problematic result. Of course, the patient doesn't always read the analyst (or the therapist) as acutely as in this example. But how the patient reads the motives of an analyst/therapist will often contribute to how the patient then experiences what follows.

Who is most helped through an analyst or therapist being helpful?

This is always an important question to ask whenever a therapist[2] moves into the mode of 'being helpful', or trying to be. As with reassurance, it is nearly always clear that the therapist *wishes* to be helpful to the patient. So why is this not always the result?

Attempts at being helpful are not always as altruistic as they may at first appear. There is often also an element of self-protection and of wanting to be seen in a good light, which is nearly always registered as such by the patient, either consciously or unconsciously. And this often seems to fit with the patient's history. So what follows may be a fusion of some external reality in the analytic relationship together with some transference elaboration based upon this. For example:

Once I had been delayed on the telephone, keeping my next patient waiting for five minutes before starting the session. When I apologized for keeping her waiting, offering extra time at the end of the session if she wished, the patient made it abundantly clear to me that she did

2 As elsewhere, I am using 'therapist' or 'analyst' to stand for either.

not want that extra time. That would not be *her* time, which had been lost and could not be reinstated. She also had no wish to 'let me off the hook' for keeping her waiting; nor did she want to give me grounds for 'feeling good at having made up the time at the end', as if there would then be no remaining issue about my lateness. In addition, she didn't want to be made to feel obligated to me for my seeing her in *my* time, to make up. The fact remained that I had not been there for her at the time agreed: I had therefore failed her in this and she had every right to be angry about it.

Comment

It was very relevant here that this patient had experienced her mother as frequently deflecting attention away from her own shortcomings, putting pressure upon the daughter to be grateful for all that her mother did for her, and to feel bad when she had sometimes dared to criticize her mother. It therefore showed significant progress in this analysis that my patient felt able to remonstrate much more freely with me, this time not allowing herself to be made to feel obligated to me, as to her mother.

So often, we find that significant others in a patient's life have been habitually driven by their own considerations, disregarding the patient and the patient's state of mind. So a patient may experience this also in relation to a therapist who tries to be helpful. *And this is not only transference*. An element of objective reality, concerning the therapist's own motivation, may have been discernible in the therapist's 'helpful' approach. So, a patient may feel that he/she is in the hands of someone who could also be acting more from self-concern than out of a more genuine concern for the patient. But, this time, there may be an opportunity to show more directly what the patient feels about it, as in this example.

However, patients are not always as direct as that patient was with me. Some patients may instead appear to be grateful, and the problem with which they have been 'helped' may appear to diminish in importance. But it is not always clear that the core of the problem has been adequately attended to, or that they have really revealed what was being felt at a deeper level. We therefore cannot rely on a patient's surface reactions to these moments of helpfulness from a therapist.

Explaining an exceptional absence

It can sometimes happen that therapists find themselves unable to keep to a fixed arrangement with a patient, and some patients can feel extremely let down by this. Usually I do not explain what is taking me away, allowing patients to have their own thoughts about this (often coloured by their own past experience) as this can lead into further useful work in the transference. But I recall one occasion when I felt that there were two particular patients who might feel seriously let down by my sudden absence (due to a funeral). I therefore felt it would be helpful if I let these two know something of *why* I would be absent. And the context here was that I had never previously been absent in this unscheduled way, other than for a day or two for illness.

To all of my other patients I simply said: 'I find that I have to be unexpectedly away next Wednesday', leaving them to imagine whatever they might. And I then found myself being accused of all manner of reasons for absenting myself: that I was not genuinely concerned for my patients, putting my own interests before them; that I was finding something more rewarding to do; that I was finding the work too much, *five* sessions in every week with analytic patients, so going off for a midweek break, etc.

However, to the two patients who seemed to be most precarious just then, I said: 'I have a problem with next Wednesday as there is a funeral that I wish to attend.' I was careful here to keep my explanation vague, giving no indication as to how close to me the death might have been. But I chose to mention 'a funeral' in order to indicate that it was for something serious that I was going to be away from my work with these two patients, for whom a break at that time was likely to be especially difficult. Of course, this explanation was meant to be helpful. But, in the event, both of these patients felt seriously let down because of it, and for several reasons.

Hearing that I would be going to a funeral was experienced by both patients as putting a pressure on them not to make a fuss about it. They each felt (in terms of their own history) obliged to protect me, as I might be feeling upset and might be vulnerable, and they both felt that they could not be angry with me for this unusual break in the therapy week. They both, therefore, felt that it might have been preferable not to have known why I was going to miss their sessions on that day.

As it turned out, I had not made it any easier for these patients by telling them of the funeral, even though at first they had each felt grateful that I had been open with them. Instead, I had treated them as if I had my own doubts as to their inner resources had they been faced with an unexplained absence – treating them as being more precarious than they felt they were. In the end, each got angry with me for having denied them a less constrained freedom to be angry about my absence, and for treating them as less capable than they were. So, once again, the wish to be helpful had actually been counter-productive.

Some possible dynamics at times when we may most urgently wish to be helpful

What may sometimes be overlooked at times of crisis in a therapy, for instance when both therapist and patient are under considerable pressure, is that both parties want to get away from this. So when (as therapists) we offer a way to relieve the tension in some crisis *we may be doing this as much for ourselves as for the patient*. And this fact is nearly always registered at some level in a patient's mind.

A further factor at these times is that there is frequently some replay of an earlier time of crisis in the patient's life. And, when we explore the history, we often find that a parent or caregiver, when the patient was a child, had in some way failed to see the child through a time that had been experienced as unmanageable. Therefore, whatever had then been unmanageable to the child may have been experienced as also being beyond the parent or caregiver's capacity to manage. Consequently, the combined effect of this can be that the child is left with an experience that is now felt to be beyond the capacity of *anyone* to tolerate or to manage.

Consequently, when such a time of early trauma is re-presented in the course of therapy, it is of central importance that the therapist be experienced as able to manage what had not previously been regarded as manageable. And this often means going through a period in the therapy that is felt to have the same quality of being unmanageable, as had been associated with that early experience.

What, therefore, are the unconscious implications for the patient when the therapist behaves in a way that seems to confirm the toxicity of some apparently unmanageable experience? I am again reminded of what Bion has said about this. For it can result in a patient again feeling, as in childhood, that he/she is left with the *nameless dread* that Bion speaks of in his paper 'A theory of thinking'. In that he says:

> If the infant feels that it is dying it can arouse fears that it is dying in the mother. A well-balanced mother can accept these and respond therapeutically: that is to say in a manner that makes the infant feel it is receiving its frightened personality back again but in a form that it can tolerate – the fears are manageable by the infant personality. If the mother cannot tolerate these projections, the infant is reduced to continued projective identification carried out with increasing force and frequency.

> (Bion, 1967: 114–115)

He later adds:

> If the projection is not accepted by the mother the infant feels that its
> feeling that it is dying is stripped of such meaning as it has. It
> therefore reintrojects, not a fear of dying made tolerable, but a
> nameless dread.
>
> (Bion, 1967: 118)

The patient will often see the therapist who offers some exceptional
way out of an intolerable situation in the therapy as having deflected the
worst in the experience that was being re-presented in the transference.
And this deflection is often felt to confirm a sense of something in that
experience as also being unmanageable for the therapist. The result of
such a manoeuvre, if followed with a discerning eye, can frequently be
seen to be twofold.

On the surface it could seem that the patient has really been helped.
The crisis may seem to have passed. The tensions that had been intolerable
might seem to have subsided. The patient appears to be grateful and may
speak of the therapist in glowing terms, even as having helped in ways
that no one else had helped. And, superficially, this could be so.

At another level, it can also be that the patient has now moved into
protecting the analyst/therapist from whatever had seemed to be too much
to bear. So, instead of risking this new and important relationship with
the therapist, the patient may become phobic of the situation that seemed
to have so nearly wrecked it. Whatever had contributed to an experience
becoming intolerable might now be kept firmly split off, displaced
elsewhere or returned to repression, safely away from the therapeutic
relationship – now seen as less resilient than it could have been without
the defensive manoeuvre in question.

An extended clinical example

A patient had returned to resume the work that we had begun in his earlier
analysis with me, which had ended nearly five years before. When Mr T
had ended that analysis, then in his early thirties, we both felt that
significant progress had been made and that he was ready to end. There
had been no feeling then of there being a *flight into health*, the patient in
any recognizable sense avoiding something in the analysis. Instead, the
ending had seemed appropriate at the time. However, just before writing
to ask if he could come back to see me, Mr T had a dream in which '*an
old wound had opened up, requiring further medical attention*'. He took

this as an unconscious sign that there was more work to be done: that some important matter(s) had not been sufficiently dealt with in the earlier analysis.

Some history

Mr T was the child of an agoraphobic mother, and one of the reasons for his coming into analysis had been his own travel phobia, he being required to travel quite a lot for his work. He had previously coped with this travelling – up to a point – by having clear limits and boundaries to where he felt able to go. But he had usually felt extreme anxiety if he ever had to go beyond those limits. However, by the time he ended that analysis with me he had become much freer to travel. And the anxiety about this, which before had been so troublesome, had become a great deal more manageable.

Mr T was the first of two children, his mother having given birth to another son when he had been aged four and a half. His mother had died of a heart attack when Mr T had been in his twenties, a death he had anticipated for most of his life, as his mother had often told him she was sure she was going to die young. He knew that he had found her death, when it actually happened, extremely difficult to cope with.

Since ending his analysis, Mr T's wife had been diagnosed as having a similar heart condition, but he had been able not to get into high anxiety over this and she had responded well to treatment. However, when he had the dream that brought him back into treatment, Mr T had understood this to be indicating that he hadn't sufficiently dealt with the death of his mother, having been so clearly reminded of this through his wife's illness.

The resumed analysis

Some months into this resumed analysis (my patient now seeing me three times per week) I had to be away for two Friday afternoons, which meant that I would have to miss seeing him on those days. And I was particularly concerned about this break in continuity so soon after his return to analysis. Alternatively, we might be able to find a replacement time for those sessions. With some difficulty Mr T found that, if he rearranged his schedule, he could come early on those two Fridays. It then looked as if his pattern of sessions would not have to be interrupted by my absence on those two days.

However, when it came to the first of these changed times, I learned from Mr T that he had been held up by 'horrendous traffic' on the way, which he never encountered when he came at his usual time. He had then re-experienced some of the acute travel anxiety that he thought he had got free of in his previous analysis with me. But I noticed that, instead of being angry with me about the change of time, he was blaming himself for having agreed to it. Eventually, he said: 'It would have been a lot better if I had just missed the session rather than trying to find another time.' He added that he anyhow prefers 'a structure which remains the same and reliable'. Now, with these two times changed, he felt 'at sea and insecure'.

Comment

My concern to make up the missed sessions was not turning out to be as helpful as I had wished. I was also to find, as the therapy continued, that Mr T was coming to see these changes as being more for *me* than they had been for *him*.

Until now Mr T had been exploring the parallels between his wife's recent diagnosis and his mother's heart condition and death. But after this time he began to be flooded with memories from around the time that his brother had been born. He recalled his parents telling him he was going on a 'nice holiday' with his grandparents. 'But', he said, 'they hadn't been honest with him.' He now felt they were getting him out of the way, and this so-called holiday had really been to suit themselves. He added: '*They hadn't done it for me at all!*' And when he got to his grandparents, he had experienced them as completely out of touch with what he was feeling, trying to divert him with activities which they assumed he was enjoying.

Mr T then recalled that there was no way he could enjoy those diversions provided by his grandparents, as he (aged four and a half) had been worried out of his mind about his mother, particularly as he knew she was going to be in a hospital. And Mr T had come to associate hospitals with people dying, his mother having already made him anxious that she could die. So, his grandparents' attempts to keep him amused, in order to distract him, had only left him feeling even more isolated with his worries.

It was becoming clear that Mr T had been experiencing me as moving his session time around to suit *myself*. Like his parents, I had presented these changes as being for *his* benefit 'to preserve the continuity of his sessions'. But as it had turned out, these changes had merely thrown him into a whole string of other difficulties. He had to rearrange his schedule in order to come at the earlier times, and then he had been caught in a terrible journey through the rush hour.

Comment

What was now emerging in Mr T's relationship to me was a strong sense of replay of the traumatic time around his brother's birth, and for a while it seemed as if this could seriously threaten the analysis. In his mind, I had become a close replica of the parents who had sent him away at a time when he was especially needy of his mother. They had also claimed that this had been for *his* sake when it had really been for *theirs*. So, in many senses I had fallen into a re-enactment of that traumatic time in his childhood. And much of it seemed to be just the same.

Gradually, however, it became apparent to Mr T that there was *one* respect in which things were different with me.

Mr T had experienced his mother as unable to cope with his upset feelings. Repeatedly, when he had shown her that he was upset about something, she seemed to become unable to cope. In the end he had learned to protect her from any upset feelings, and in particular his anger. It was only with people he didn't know, as in a shop, that he could let himself be as angry as he felt, as when something had gone wrong that shouldn't. Then, the anger that poured out of him was often quite alarming: to himself as well as to the person on the receiving end of it.

Now, at this moment in the therapy, Mr T had found that my attempt at being helpful had not helped him at all. *It had only helped me*, as it had given me a chance not to feel so bad about my being away on those two Friday afternoons. In a real sense, therefore, he could feel completely justified in being angry with me – as with a shop assistant when something had gone wrong. But the anger he felt towards me also had its roots in his early relationship to his parents, and especially his mother.

The specific difference that Mr T began to find, between his mother and me, was as follows. Whereas his mother could not bear him to be angry with her, he came to realize that I was actually 'there' for his anger. And, for a while, I was taking this anger as if it were *not* transference but as just for me. Then, as his associations led us back to the time when he had been sent away, while his mother was giving birth to his brother, he began to use me to represent the mother of that time. He could remember feeling *extremely* upset and angry with her then, but he had not been able to express any of that to her. He now found he had become able to give a much more direct expression of those feelings to me, using me to represent the mother who had sent him away.

Moreover, finding he had this valid occasion for his anger towards me, he also began to get in touch with that other anger which had remained for so long locked into his unconscious mind. There we began to find that *nameless dread* (associated with this anger) which had resulted from his mother seeming to be unable to bear being properly in touch with his most difficult feelings.

Maybe we had reached the 'old wound' which Mr T had dreamed of, returning to see me for this to receive the further attention that had been missing in his earlier analysis, and for it now to begin to heal. (For what still lay ahead in this analysis, see the following chapter.)

Conclusion

What I have tried to illustrate here, in this vignette from my work with Mr T, is that we can all too easily delude ourselves around the issue of 'being helpful' in psychotherapy. We may quite frequently aim at being helpful, and our patients may reward our attempts as if they have been helped, but at another level there could be something quite different that is going on.

Most particularly when a patient has been traumatized we will frequently find that the patient brings into the analytic relationship key aspects of that trauma for reworking. There will always have been strong feelings at a time of trauma, and it has often been the case that there had been no one there to help with those feelings. And, let us remember, one of the characteristics of early trauma is that it could not be adequately managed alone.

Clinical experience bears out that what is most helpful to patients, in the long term, is not necessarily to be found through a therapist offering to be 'better' than those who had previously let them down. A patient who has been traumatized needs, above all else, to discover that the worst within the internal world of the mind, which others had not been able to bear, *can* be managed within the analytic relationship. And this essentially involves the 'worst' in the patient's life being brought into the analytic relationship, being re-experienced there – even re-enacted there, in order to find a containment of this 'worst' that had not formerly been found.

A turning point towards a real recovery, not based upon avoidance, may then grow out of such times of pain that are genuinely borne and lived through by the therapist and patient together. The result then may be something very different from those other times when the therapist has steered the therapy into 'quieter waters'.

Chapter 6

Re-enactment and resolution

An extraordinary clinical finding is that we sometimes succeed in analysis when it seems that we are most especially failing.

Introduction

Winnicott was probably the first to observe that we sometimes succeed by failing. Of this he said:

> The corrective provision is never enough. What is it that may be enough for some of our patients to get well? In the end the patient uses the analyst's failures, often quite small ones, perhaps manoeuvred by the patient, or the patient produces delusional transference elements (Little, 1958) and we have to put up with being in a limited context misunderstood. The operative factor is that the patient now hates the analyst for the failure that originally came as an environmental factor, outside the infant's area of omnipotent control, but that is now staged in the transference.
>
> So in the end we succeed by failing – failing the patient's way.
>
> (Winnicott, 1963b: 344)

What I may need to stress, before proceeding to the clinical material in this chapter, is that I found myself making some quite extraordinary mistakes in the sequence I shall describe. At first glance it might look as if I was merely being careless or inattentive. And I have to agree that there must have been some element of both operating at the time. And yet, the strange fact is that I was most particularly concerned *not* to be letting down this patient during his renewed analysis. So how could it have happened? I am still having to wonder about that. An equally important question is how could this have turned out to have become a positive turning point in the overall analysis of this patient?[1]

There are times when, despite our own conscious intentions, we can be drawn into a dynamic with a particular patient that is 'beyond our ken'. Sandler was speaking of this when he wrote:

> Parallel to the 'free-floating attention' of the analyst is what I should like to call his free-floating responsiveness. The analyst is, of course, not a machine in absolute self-control, only experiencing on the one hand, and delivering interpretations on the other, although much of the literature might seem to paint such a picture. Among many other things he talks, he greets the patient, he makes arrangements about practical matters, he may joke and, to some degree, allow his responses to depart from the classical psychoanalytic norm. My contention is that in the analyst's overt reactions to the patient as well as in his thoughts and feelings what can be called his 'role-responsiveness' shows itself, not only in his feelings but also in his attitudes and behaviour, as a crucial element in his 'useful' countertransference.
>
> (Sandler, 1976: 45)

Let us continue now with the case described in Chapter 5, following some more of that patient's search for the analytic experience that was still eluding both him and me.

The case

From the previous analysis

In the course of Mr T's initial analysis with me I had learned much about his early childhood. In particular, a key trauma in his life had been around the fact that his maternal grandmother had died *on the same day that he was born*. This meant that his own mother was caught between the two experiences of death and birth (see Lewis and Casement, 1986), unable

---

1 I do not share with Renik the view that enactments are necessary to an analysis, even if they are inevitable (Renik, 1993). I believe that enactments by the analyst can be very destructive to an analysis and are, as far as possible, to be avoided. A great deal therefore depends upon how a patient views an enactment and how it comes to be used. On this Chused writes: 'A patient's understanding of an enactment within the analytic relationship will be determined by the patient's psychic reality, by how he perceives and understands the analyst's behavior, not by the analyst's understanding of the enactment' (1997: 268).

to deal adequately with either because of these occurring together. This inability seems to have resulted in her failing to mourn that death, and equally failing to celebrate her son's birth. So, Mr T found himself being nursed by a depressed and anxious mother, who may well have found it difficult to be truly *present* to him, emotionally, or to be responsively available.

At the age of four and half Mr T had the double upset of not only being displaced by his brother's birth but also being sent off to infant school very soon after it. The apparent reason for the decision to send him to school so early seems to have been that his father saw the mother as not able to cope with two children all day, she (being anxious and agoraphobic) now having her hands full with this new baby.

During his early years, Mr T had come to see his mother as quite seriously fragile. Not only could she barely cope with any travelling, even at home she was often seriously anxious. And, in particular, he registered that she seemed to be barely able to cope with any distress from him when he was upset. In fact, Mr T learned to watch his mother very closely for any signs of anxiety, lest he might further upset her. And his own anxiety about this was brought even more strongly to a focus when someone else's mother, only two doors away, had committed suicide. He had been told something of this, in terms of the neighbour having found life too difficult, which fed into his anxiety that his mother might also find life too much if he failed to protect her sufficiently from his own upset feelings and difficulties.

Mr T came to feel that it was *his* responsibility to make his mother better whenever she became upset. And, even from a young age, he used to be the one member of the family who seemed to be able to deal with her when she had shut herself in her room, crying. He would knock on the door, pleading to be allowed in, so that he could comfort her and make her better. In many respects, he virtually became a little mother (or even a little therapist) to his own mother.

When Mr T was old enough for primary school education, his father decided that his son should not be sent to the school nearby, apparently thinking that it would have been too easy for the boy to come home if he didn't like it. Also, he would have been able to come home for lunch each day. That might either have been too much for the mother, or the father seemed to think that it would not be good for the boy to remain so close to home. Being sent further away 'might stop him becoming a mother's boy', this being one of the father's concerns.

The journey to and from that school became a great trial for Mr T. On his return journey he would sometimes have to wait for nearly an hour for a bus that was not full up, before he was allowed to travel home, and he also had to negotiate a change of buses *en route*. As he remembers it, he used to worry all the way home about how his mother would be when he got back, particularly if his journey had been delayed. And the more anxious he was during this journey the more strongly did he feel he had to conceal any sign of this from his mother when he got home, in order not to upset her. In effect, he had to 'mother' himself. And he remembered a ritual, always observed as he neared his home, in which he would actively try to get rid of his anxiety before seeing his mother. He knew that he could not completely get rid of this, but he remembers working on himself to conceal any visible evidence of his having been upset before he got home.

By the time he first came to see me, Mr T had developed a serious travel problem of his own, which superficially seemed to be in identification with his claustrophobic mother. But we soon came to see that there were other factors in this that were much more specific to himself. For instance, Mr T discovered he could only travel away from home if he knew where he could find a toilet along the route of his journey, in case he urgently needed this.

During his earlier analysis with me, Mr T managed to push at the boundaries of his travel areas so that he gradually became able to undertake journeys which had before seemed impossible for him. But he had continued to have a serious anxiety about being 'caught short' at a time when he might not have immediate access to a toilet. However, what began to make sense of this *conversion symptom*, as we came to understand it, was that Mr T was still feeling a need to get rid of difficult feelings, as if he still had to 'protect the mother in his mind' from anything that could be upsetting to her. So the more anxious he became, the more he felt he had to get rid of this anxiety, symbolically, through evacuation.

We then came to a crucial time that I have described elsewhere,[2] during which Mr T became increasingly able to trust me with what he was feeling. These feelings no longer had to be regarded as dangerous, having to be got rid of down toilets in the form of faeces. Instead, his upset feelings could be brought to me in the analysis and they could be allowed direct expression, such as he had never felt able to show to his mother. And his symptoms began to disappear.

---

2 This has been published in *Further Learning from the Patient* (Casement, 1990: Chapter 10, example 10.4) and *Learning from the Patient* (Casement, 1991: Chapter 20, example 20.4) but, for the sake of the thesis of this chapter, I repeat a part of that here.

Mr T then became able to manage journeys that he had never thought possible before, and he could travel without needing to check on the availability of toilets. His feelings also began to be experienced as communicable, and as manageable by another. And he no longer had to attempt to be 'his own mother'. Neither did he still have to protect the mother in his mind; nor, in the transference, did he feel he had to protect me as that mother.

Mr T gradually began to feel that he had achieved what he had aimed for in his analysis, and a lot more than he had dared to hope for. So, around four and a half years from the beginning of his analysis Mr T had left, feeling much better.

With hindsight, however, we eventually came to see that the main benefit for Mr T from that first period of analysis had been through his discovery that I had been better able to attend to his emotional needs than his mother had seemed to be. But this had not been enough, as was indicated by the dream that brought him back to analysis.

The renewed analysis

I shall now describe some more of what happened in this follow-up analysis. As mentioned in Chapter 5, Mr T had asked to come back into analysis after the dream in which *he had found an old wound opening up and requiring further treatment.* He was now coming three days a week: Wednesday, Thursday and Friday.

In this renewed analysis, Mr T had been finding his way to express much more directly to me the feelings which he had not been able to express to his mother (see Chapter 5), and which we had not got to in that earlier analysis. But there was yet more to come.

Some practical details

Patients who arrive early for a session use my waiting room, where there are several chairs. Most sit far into the room, which means that I have to walk some way in before I can greet them. Mr T, however, would always sit in a chair directly facing the door. Usually, patients (including Mr T) would leave the door nearly closed. I therefore need to be mindful of which patient I am about to collect from the waiting room as it makes a difference to how I open the door: whether to remain in the doorway for a patient using the chair opposite (as for Mr T), or whether to stride into the room for a patient sitting further into it.

Then, when coming into my consulting room, my patients go in first and I follow, firmly shutting each of the two doors as I come in. Usually the patient starts getting onto the couch (which faces the door) while I walk to my chair at the head of the couch.

Some patients expect me to place a tissue on the pillow. A few patients, like Mr T, are used to having the pillow *without* a tissue.[3] So, once again, I had to keep in mind which patient I was expecting so that the couch was appropriately prepared.

Going to collect a different patient

On a Wednesday, immediately prior to one of Mr T's sessions, I had been waiting for the previous patient who had not come. Then, when Mr T arrived for his session, I was still mentally prepared for that previous patient, *not Mr T*. So, when I went to the waiting room, thinking that I was about to collect someone else, I strode into the room as I would for her. To my surprise, I found that I had stepped up towards Mr T, who was sitting as usual opposite the door. He obviously noticed that I was 'on the wrong foot' when I got into the room. Then, when Mr T went into the consulting room, it became even more clear that I had been expecting someone different. The pillow on the couch had remained as for the previous patient, who (unlike Mr T) was used to having a tissue on the pillow.

I was particularly shocked by this mistake, as I had done exactly the same thing a few weeks before. So, as I went to remove the tissue, I said (with an anxious laugh) '*I've done it again*', this being already the second time I had made this same mistake. Mr T also laughed and my mistakes were not referred to again in that session, by him or by me.

During that session, I was looking for some way to pick up an allusion to these mistakes, in what Mr T was saying. However, either there were none or I was failing to notice them. But there was also a further problem. Due to my haste in going to remove the tissue, the inner door to my consulting room (which opens away from the couch) had slipped open again after I thought that I had closed it. And I only noticed this later.

Once I had noticed the door, I had hoped that when Mr T made some reference to this repeating of my earlier confusion, over which patient I

---

3 The background to my allowing each patient to choose whether to have a tissue on the pillow, or not, goes back to my own therapy and subsequent analysis. Neither my therapist nor my analyst provided tissues for the pillow, and for many years neither did I. Eventually, however, a few patients asked for this, which then resulted in my practice of providing each patient with what he/she had been used to or had expressed a wish for. I tried to remain consistent with each patient individually, but on this occasion I was failing in this.

was expecting, I could have included a reference to the inner door not being firmly closed. (I had thought that it would be less intrusive if I had got up to close it once we were addressing the problem of these mistakes than doing so earlier on.) However, Mr T had apparently not noticed this so I thought it might not be disturbing him as much it was disturbing me, and I knew that the outside door was definitely closed. With hindsight, I could recognize that I was also wanting to hide my embarrassment over having also 'messed up' over the door. All in all, I was into an extraordinary degree of distraction, and of enactment, which at the time I could not understand.

The next day, Mr T started by saying that he had left yesterday's session with a headache and it had persisted throughout the day. In fact there was still something of this around today. He then went on to say he thought it may have been to do with something that happened during the day, and he went into some details about his wife's visit to the doctor. She had gone for a further check-up on her heart condition. But Mr T had 'for some reason' completely forgotten to ask her about it when he got home in the evening. He had then felt terrible about this, as soon as he had remembered, and he had wondered whether it had been due to his anxiety about her check-up that he had gone around for much of the day with the headache that he had mentioned.

At this point, I said: 'There certainly does seem to have been something that upset you yesterday.' [I was choosing to keep it open, for Mr T to make his own link to the previous session – if he did.]

Mr T then told me a dream in which *he had come for his session but he had found that the couch had been moved over to another corner of the room. Things were just not the same.*

In exploring this dream, Mr T's associations led back to the time when his mother had said to him that 'everything would be just the same' after his brother had been born. But things had actually been completely different. He had discovered that his mother seemed to be principally concerned with the new baby while he felt he had been left to manage largely on his own.

I then pointed out that it was not difficult to see connections here to the previous session, when I had someone else in mind before the start of the session. Mr T picked this up, agreeing with me, and went on to point out that there was also something else that was wrong with the previous session. He said that I might not have noticed it, and he would have been surprised if I *had* noticed as he had only made a 'token protest' about it at the end of the session. But, when he had left he had found the inner door not properly closed. Usually, when he leaves, he shuts the inner door and leaves the outer door ajar. But, yesterday, he had left the *inner* door ajar (as he had found it) and had closed the *outer* door. He explained that this had been his way of protesting about the inner door having been left open, in leaving it exactly as it had been during the session – not quite closed.

I commented on the indirectness of this communication, as with his mother, as if I might not have been able to bear a more direct confrontation about it. Mr T agreed and reminded me of a picture book he had made, when he was five, which he had deliberately not given to his mother but had given to the little girl next door, as if to point out that the girl was being preferred over his mother.

Mr T then remembered two other 'enacted communications' to his mother, which she either failed to understand or had never talked about. One example (again when he was about five) was that he used to hide a piece of his mother's jewellery, so that she would find it had disappeared. She would then get upset about losing it, or not being able to find it, until he would eventually let her know where he had hidden it. He felt sure she must have realized that this was his way of indicating to her that he was unhappy about something, but *she never picked up the communication in this*.

Another pattern in his childhood, which we had been discussing in the previous week, was that Mr T had noticed he had repeatedly 'made friends with only children', inviting each one in turn to become his friend, and then he would drop them. He counted up a surprising number of these children, to whom he had seemed to offer to be a special friend. But he had always ended up becoming tired of them and dropping them, each time with the child feeling very hurt. Again, his mother seemed never to have recognized what was being enacted in this repeating pattern. Each time there had been *an only child, who had been led to feel he was special but who had then come to be dropped and shut out*. He pointed out that this so exactly described his own situation with his mother.

In the analytic work that followed this we came to see some striking parallels. The pattern he had been remembering had come to be re-enacted in his relationship to me. Due to some preoccupation of my own, not directly to do with Mr T, I had let him drop out of my mind at a crucial time. And I had already done this more than once. There must have been some unconscious communication here (at least in terms of personal countertransference), in my forgetting him and having the consulting room prepared for someone else, but this had been pushed to one side on the first occasion (a few weeks before). In this being repeated it had become an even more urgent matter that I reflect on this, and that we also attend to what this had come to represent to Mr T. It became evident that the problem he had so often *talked about*, in relation to his mother, had mistakenly come to be *re-enacted* by me.

In the last session of this week Mr T came back to the open door. He had left the Wednesday session thinking I had not realized the inner door had been left open. He could see how this had happened, in that I had hurried across to the couch to remove the tissue, but he felt sure I would have closed the door if I had known it had been open. And he too had not seen this until he had left the session. So, he had thought (during the Wednesday session) that it might have been something embarrassing for him, as well as for me, if he got round to pointing out that I had also overlooked the door. But then I had confessed to having seen the door partly open. *So, how was it I had done nothing about it?* This seemed to make me even more like his mother and her not seeing the meaning, as in the repeated situations he had been reminding me of (mentioned above). He had been acting out something against those only children, doing to them what he felt his mother had done to him. After all, she had dropped him (who until then had been her only child) for someone else – his brother. And I had now done this too.

Mr T's headache therefore seemed to have been something quite different from what he had first thought. Even though he was also worrying about his wife's check-up, and he had been attacking himself for not having remembered to ask her about it as soon as he got back, there was surely another dimension to it. He had almost certainly got into some of that earlier anger towards me, as a reminder of his mother who had seemed not to keep him enough in mind when his brother was born. I had done something so exactly parallel to that, *in not keeping him enough in mind*.

As we looked further into what had been happening, it became obvious that Mr T had sensed my embarrassment over it. And, again just like his mother, I had deflected his upset about this with my embarrassed laugh. So of course Mr T could experience me as just like his mother who, also in very slight ways, seems to have indicated when she had a problem with his upset feelings. And he had learned to protect her. So Mr T had been protecting me on the Wednesday, in that he had made no reference to how the session had started, and I had failed to see allusions to this in his silence about it.

We can now see that there were quite a number of striking parallels here to key issues between Mr T and his mother, particularly around the time of his brother's birth. And it is extraordinary that the re-enactment was so complete. But I believe this happens more often than we like to admit to ourselves (or to others). And yet, even though it offers no justification, at times like this there may be an unconscious resonance between the analyst and what has been the patient's history, whereby enactments bring into the analytic relationship primary aspects of problems that the patient has experienced before. And, through this, the patient may then discover the right to be as angry as may be, in a situation where this cannot be passed off as 'just' transference. I think that this is what Winnicott was speaking of, as in the quotation with which I began this chapter.

So far in this further analysis we had been able to see how I had repeated key aspects of his experience with his mother, whereby his feelings about her had come to be experienced directly in relation to me. But what was still missing was a truly unrestrained expression of Mr T's feelings about these enactments, expressed directly to me.

Naturally, I had given a lot of thought to what had been happening in these recent weeks, particularly as I had already repeated this pattern of mistakes. But, however difficult it is to explain, and it certainly cannot be explained away, this sequence happened *yet one more time*.

One Thursday, a few weeks later, I was again caught up with something that had preoccupied me while I was waiting for Mr T. I then suddenly noticed that the cushion on the couch had no tissue on it. So I put a tissue in place, as I would for the patient who (on Thursdays) came *after* Mr T. But it was once again not her time. It was his!

When the session was due to begin I went (as before) to the waiting room, still thinking that I was going to meet this other patient.[4] Once again, now the third time, I strode into the waiting room, as I would to fetch that other patient, only to find Mr T sitting on his usual chair opposite to the door. I immediately knew that he had noticed, and I burst out with: 'My God! I have done it *yet again!*'

Mr T came into the consulting room, thinking that I had merely walked into the waiting room in the wrong way, as before. But, once again, there was a tissue on the pillow! This now was a moment of acute crisis, and I realized there was a considerable risk that the analytic work with this patient could be destroyed by this. His trust in me might never recover. So it was not at all surprising that Mr T was extremely angry with me for the duration of this Thursday session. And there was no place whatever

---

4 This other patient was the same one on each of these occasions, who happened to be missing sessions around that time. Although I continued to be concerned not to let down Mr T, my attention was being deflected from him by my concern over this other patient's absences.

for any attempt (by me) at interpreting this as transference. It was with *me* that he was angry and I had to accept all of this as meant for me. *How could I have let it happen a third time?* This was a question I was asking myself just as much as he was demanding that I should explain how this had come to happen. It was beyond belief that I could have done this yet again; and I really felt it was completely unforgivable.

During this session we came to see how different it was from the previous two times. The first occasion had been brushed aside by Mr T as if it had been an easy mistake to make. The second time it had been defensively played down by me, in my laughing at myself and thereby inviting him to laugh too. But now there was no way that any of this could be brushed aside.

However, what was new on this occasion was that I had not been waiting for a patient who hadn't come (the patient before him on the Wednesday). On this Thursday I had been waiting for someone who was due to come *after* him, and I had told him this during the session.

This new detail brought about very strong associations to Mr T's brother, the one who came after him, and he spoke of the tissue as a 'towel'. When I pointed this out to him he told me it was in fact strangely close to the facts of his childhood, as his mother had not had the old type of rough nappies for his brother, but a smooth kind of towel nappy, rather like the tissue on the pillow. But, even though some connection to his history had been made, in this reference to the tissue as a towel, the focus throughout the session was upon his utter disbelief that I could have let this happen a third time.

The next day (the Friday), Mr T did not come and I spent a very uncomfortable time, knowing that this had to be because of my repeated mistake on the previous day. Mr T had never before missed an entire session without telephoning to let me know something had prevented him. On this Friday, not only was he absent but so was his usual telephone call. I therefore spent the full 50 minutes attending to Mr T's absence, and my shocking contribution to it. I felt that I might never see him again. And if I didn't I would only have myself to blame.

After I had started my next session of that day, Mr T left a message on my answerphone, letting me know that he had run into heavy traffic so that he had decided to go back home. (His journey to me was long.) It was only on the Wednesday of the following week that Mr T told me he could have got to his session. But, as the traffic was going to make the time short, he had decided early in his journey to go back home. He had also decided, quite deliberately, that he would not telephone me until he was sure I would be engaged with my next patient. He definitely didn't want to speak to me.

Mr T was determined not to do anything that could seem to smooth over the problem between us, or to lessen his anger towards me. And he most definitely wanted me to know it had been his *choice* not to come, and he wanted me to have that thought to consider over the weekend. He also didn't want to leave me with any reason to ring him. If I had not heard from him I might then have intruded into his weekend by telephoning to check whether he was all right.

So, as Mr T made very clear to me, *he had deliberately used his session that way, by not coming and by not phoning until later*. He had wanted me to feel the full force of his anger and he wanted me to have to deal with that in myself, right through from the Friday until his next session, which would not be until the following Wednesday. And he certainly succeeded in that.

What came out of this third time of my making this series of mistakes was the fullest expression ever of Mr T's anger towards me, including his use of the Friday session by not coming. And this was the kind of anger he had never been able to express to his mother, or to anyone who mattered to him. In fact, he had only ever been able to be that angry before when it was to people more remote from him, an intense anger that felt (to him) to be *lethal* because it felt so murderous. And he used to worry that his mother might die if he had ever got really angry with her.

Mr T knew without a doubt that I had felt the impact of this 'white hot anger'. But what had been most important to him had been that I had been willing to be 'there' for it. This time I had not brushed any of it aside, and neither had he. His anger was there in all its force. But he also began to feel a confidence that I could bear it. And throughout his weekend, after the missed session, he had not been at all anxious. Previously, with his mother, he had constantly felt he had to check that she was surviving, that she was not being made upset by his being upset, or by the possibility that he might be angry with her. But, with me, he had felt entirely all right about being as angry with me as he had been, and still was. He also felt quietly confident that I would be able to take it, so that he had not worried about this at any stage during the weekend.

Not long after this I had to cancel two sessions in order to have some minor surgery. Because of the slight chance of complications, which could have resulted in my having to remain in hospital for two or three weeks, I chose to let Mr T know the reason for my absence. What then was interesting, and significant, was that he was able to be entirely relaxed about this over the intervening time until his next session. He told me later that he knew I would have let him know if there had been any problem. So, not hearing from me meant that all must be well and he could wait until his next session without becoming anxious about my well-being. This, coming soon after he had been so angry with me, was something entirely new for him. And this seemed to have grown out of a new confidence that his anger, after all, did not still have to be regarded as harmful, let alone as lethal, as it had for so long seemed to be.

Discussion

In this sequence I have wanted to show how, as part of the analytic process, patients may revisit key experiences of early failure by their parents, or other caregivers, through their use of similar failures by the analyst.

How much this discovered similarity in an analysis is fortuitous, and how much it may be unconsciously determined, we may never quite know (cf. Winnicott, 1958: Chapter 22; 1965b: Chapter 23). But it can be quite uncanny to what extent a patient can find such opportunities for trans-ference, by means of which key experiences from the past are then relived in relation to the analyst. Together with this, I believe there can be an *unconscious hope*[5] of being able to find help in dealing differently with those earlier experiences, and in working them through in the analysis.

I had failed Mr T in a most significant way. And I had continued to fail him until the repeated re-enactment resulted in a major change in his relating to me. I could never justify such a degree of failure as this, and I still feel shocked that I could have remained caught into this as long as I did. But, at the same time, it is strange how precisely we can fail some patients, in ways that really do seem to be 'determined by' their history, as Winnicott describes. It was as if I was being caught into a different state of consciousness, around the time of Mr T's sessions, until we got to where we did. And it was only after this that he began to feel that we had got to where we needed to, in particular to 'the wound that had not healed' that had brought him back into analysis, and for this to receive the further healing which had been so necessary.

In the analytic relationship, particularly in the first period of the analysis, Mr T appeared to find in me a 'better mother', in that he felt I had been able to be better in touch with his distress than his mother seems to have been. But when Mr T came back for this further period of analysis it was he who pointed out to me that it may have been no coincidence he

---

5 I have discussed this notion of unconscious hope at some length elsewhere (Casement, 1990: Chapter 7; 1991: Chapter 17).

had left the earlier analysis when he did: after four and a half years. It was true he had made significant progress in that analysis, but he had only later noticed that he had been in analysis with me for almost exactly the same amount of time he had been with his mother before his brother was born. He strongly agreed with me when I said: 'Maybe you left while the going was good.'

After almost exactly the same amount of time away from his analysis (another four and a half years) Mr T began to recognize that his progress had not been maintained. Some of his symptoms had returned. He then had the dream about the wound that needed further attention, leading to his letter asking me if he could come back into treatment.

As described in Chapter 5, at the time of his writing to me Mr T had thought he might be needing to do further analytic work around his mother's death, his wife's illness having brought this back to him very directly. But, once he had restarted his sessions with me, it had very quickly become apparent that the unworked-through trauma had been more to do with the events around the birth of his brother, which he had then begun to remember and to re-experience.

Then, through the sequence in this present chapter, Mr T found a way into expressing his most extreme anger *directly* at me – his anger now being fully justified. And, however strange it might seem to the reader, Mr T actually felt a relief resulting from this: a relief that had eluded him throughout all of our other analytic work together.

Some readers might conclude that, when my patient came to leave this renewed period of analysis, it might have been to protect himself from an analyst who could be so seriously unmindful of him as to have been repeatedly thinking of some other patient. And I have had to ask myself that too. But, in the remaining time of this further analysis, Mr T became convinced that we had now got to what had previously been insufficiently attended to.

Here was the wound which had needed further attention. Here was the anger that had always felt so dangerous to him (even lethal). And this was no longer being kept away from me, as it had been throughout the time when he had experienced me as being 'better than' his parents, and in particular his mother. It was through his using me to represent the key *failure(s)* experienced with his mother that he had found release. He now was able to move on from his life-long conviction that no one would be able to bear the intensity of his anger and his upset.

Mr T had needed me to be 'there' for that anger, and that upset, and for me not to be protecting myself with any transference interpretations. Only then could we also attend to his transference use of me, as he had come to experience me during that sequence. So, as Winnicott had recognized in his own clinical work, I too had succeeded by failing my patient – in ways so precisely parallel to those times when he had experienced the most difficulty. It then became possible for my failure here to be turned to positive use, through my being present and willing to go through the fullest expression of his most intense feelings and transference in response to this. And it is here, in particular, that we find that which goes beyond any attempt at *corrective emotional experience* (Alexander *et al.*, 1946).

Yet again, it is not by being a 'better parent' that we are able to deal with the deepest effects of early trauma. It is by being there for a patient's most difficult feelings, often associated with trauma and seeming to have been more than others could bear, that a patient can eventually find experience that *is* better and that is healing.

I return to this theme in the next chapter.

Chapter 7

To hold or not to hold a patient's hand: further reflections

What ultimately proves to be most therapeutic may often lie far beyond our own imagination or devising.

Is physical contact with the patient, even of a token kind, always to be precluded without question under the classical rule of abstinence? Or are there some occasions when this might be appropriate, even necessary, as Margaret Little has suggested in relation to episodes of delusional transference or as Balint and Winnicott have illustrated in relation to periods of deep regression?

(Casement, 1982: 279)

It is now twenty years since I wrote my paper 'Some pressures on the analyst for physical contact during the reliving of an early psychic trauma', which was first presented at the Helsinki Congress of the IPA and subsequently published in the *International Review of Psycho-Analysis* (Casement, 1982).[1]

For some reason this paper has remained the focus of much discussion, some of it quite heated, so it seems appropriate to be returning to this now as it illustrates so specifically the issues being discussed in this book. This continuing discussion also has more general relevance, as it touches on issues that are central to the process of psychoanalysis and, in particular, to work with patients who have been traumatized.

Amongst the unpublished discussions of this paper, either in my presence or that have been reported to me, there have been some quite

---

1 This paper was also published in Casement (1985: Chapter 7), and in Casement (1991: Chapter 7). In addition it was reprinted in Kohon (1986: 282–294).

serious criticisms of how I handled my patient (Mrs B) during the sessions that I have described. I have, for instance, been seen as having been cruel to her. And some people have seen me as being rigid, rule-bound and insensitive to my patient's needs. I have also been seen as failing to follow my patient's explicit cues. And much else. Not all discussants, however, have been unsympathetic to my handling of that case.[2]

I shall give an outline below of the paper in question, but some readers might prefer to read the original text, which can be found in the Appendix, before continuing with this chapter.

Much of the text in this chapter is extracted from 'The issue of touch: a retrospective overview' (Casement, 2000).

Background

For those not familiar with this case I shall give a few details. The patient described in this clinical presentation had been seriously scalded when she was 11 months old. At the age of 17 months she had been operated on (under local anaesthetic) to release scar tissue from the surrounding skin. During this procedure the patient's mother was holding her hand until she had fainted. In reliving this experience, of being left alone with the surgeon who continued to operate on her regardless of the mother's absence, the patient asked (and later demanded) to be allowed to hold my hand if the anxiety became intolerable to bear. If I could not agree to this she felt that she would have to terminate the analysis. In reconsidering this demand, I decided after much careful reflection that it would amount to a collusive avoidance of the central aspect of the original trauma, which had been the absence of the mother's hands after she had fainted. But I only came to see the need to withdraw that hand-holding offer as a result of closely following the patient's unconscious communications to me (see below).

The restoration of the analytic holding,[3] without physical contact, and the eventual resolution of the near-delusional transference at this time in the analysis, is examined in detail in the original paper. The interpretation, which eventually proved effective in restoring contact with the patient's readiness to continue with her analysis, emerged from a close following

---

2 For other discussion, see also Aron (1992), Boesky (1998), Fox (1984), Hoffer (1991), Katz (1998), Meissner (1996, 1998), Roughton (1993).
3 It has been said that a patient feels most securely held in an analysis when feeling properly understood.

of my countertransference responses to the patient and what I believed to be the projective-identificatory pressures[4] upon me that I sensed during this time.

Contrary to what some people have assumed, my decision to withdraw the offer of my hand was not in any way made on the basis of any rule of abstinence. It was based on following the patient at a deeper level than just that of her surface communications to me. All of my clinical writing has been an attempt to show the importance of following the patient. So my commitment, throughout the analysis of Mrs B, was to follow (*really* follow) her overall communications, rather than being committed to any particular point of theory or technique. And when we do follow the patient's communications beyond just the manifest level of what is being asked of us, or demanded, we sometimes arrive at a position that is far less comfortable than anything we might personally have chosen.

A lot of the discussion, in *Psychoanalytic Inquiry* and elsewhere, seems either to have been based on assumptions about why I acted as I did, or to have been influenced by a lack of other clinical detail that might have provided a fuller context for further discussion. I hope now to clarify, better than I seem to have done in my original paper, the context within which all of this work was being carried out.

Further reflections on the clinical sequence under discussion

One of the main issues, during the first two years or so of this long analysis, was that Mrs B had been seriously traumatized at a time of continuing dependence. She had therefore developed the defence of 'self-holding', whereby she sought to protect herself from ever again depending on another person – at least at any deep level of dependence.

It had thus been a feature throughout those first years of her analysis that Mrs B would frequently seek to control me; a control that I initially would allow her. Latterly, however, she had begun to relax from that near total control. Occasionally, I had stood my ground in the course of some interpretive work, as when I did not accept her signal for me to stop (see

---

4 One understanding of the process of *projective identification* (Klein, 1946) is that a person who cannot bear the intensity of some feeling or distress may induce another person to experience some of this in response to interactional pressures that prompt such feelings in the other. The unconscious aim in this interactional communication seems to be either to get rid of what cannot be managed alone or to seek help with it from another person.

Appendix, p. 130). Gradually, through such moments as these, Mrs B had begun to allow me a more separate existence, with a mind of my own that was not held so totally within her control.

I believe we had to find a way for this gradual differentiation between herself and me, as not merged and as not totally controlled by her, in preparation for what was to come later. Winnicott speaks of this in his paper 'Use of an object' (Winnicott, 1971b), as a necessary step towards a patient becoming able to 'use' the analyst, who is thus found to have *a capacity to survive* which actually belongs to the object and is not merely 'given' (in phantasy) by the patient.

With some patients, this discovery alone can lead to a fuller experience of being held, when that holding truly comes from an 'other' who is no longer seen merely as an extension of the patient's own self-holding. So this was an important background to the sessions under discussion.

In the course of the session just referred to, my not stopping when Mrs B had signalled to me came to be experienced as my being too much like 'the surgeon who had carried on regardless'. This is precisely what Winnicott writes about when he says that, at a crucial moment, we will find (as already illustrated in the previous chapter) that we have failed a patient 'in ways determined by [the patient's] past history' (Winnicott, 1965b: 258–259).

Another background issue, which had been there from the beginning of this analysis but which had been coming increasingly to the fore in recent months, was Mrs B's belief that no one would be able to survive the full impact of her feelings: of her neediness, her anger, her rage and her despair. As part of her characteristic defence against this anticipated collapse of the other person, and of me as her analyst, Mrs B had frequently stayed with *relating the details* of her traumatic past as an account of her life story. For a long time, therefore, she had thus avoided *relating to me* except as to a hearer of her narrative, thus limiting her emotional and/or relationship demands upon me.

One contributor (to *Psychoanalytic Inquiry*) suggested that Mrs B would still have been able to 'talk about' her traumatic experience, even had I been holding her hand, and she might even have been better able to talk about it under those circumstances (Fosshage, 2000: 36). But a major step with regard to this had begun to be taken in her analysis, in that Mrs B had begun to relate to me more directly, with the feelings that belonged to those figures in her past who had apparently *not* survived her neediness. She no longer just 'talked about' what had happened to her. At this time in the analysis she was definitely beginning to relate more directly to me, as to a person relating to her, rather than to me as someone there just to hear her story. This, however, was bringing her into the area of her greatest fears: that I might actually collapse under the weight of her neediness. This was not only her fear: it was her *conviction* that I would collapse.

So, we come to the sessions under discussion.

On the Friday, my initial countertransference was largely governed by my fear that I might lose my patient. But I didn't feel particularly uncomfortable about the proposed handling of this – for her to have the possibility of holding my hand if it became intolerable. There had already been some analysts before me, such as Balint and Winnicott, who had found the courage to challenge the classical position. So why shouldn't I? And, surely, nobody could seriously question my decision to let this patient hold my hand, or just have the *possibility* of holding my hand, in these particular circumstances. How could anyone challenge my judgement on that, I thought, if I had kept open the offer for her to hold my hand *if necessary* – with this patient's history of a mother whose hand had slipped out of hers at such a crucial moment? And, in any case, my clinical position had long been that of a protester against any blind following of rules.

Breckenridge (2000: 7–8) says she regards it as essential for the question of touch to be considered from within one's own particular limits, suggesting that even the possibility of Mrs B holding my hand had gone beyond my personal limits. In fact, my limits had to be *extended* by the Monday in order to find the courage to go through this sequence without that. The safer course for me had been the one I was offering to take on that Friday. But, I had to find a way that went far beyond this if I were not to let down my patient.

What began to shake my almost complacent acceptance that my patient could hold my hand, if it began to feel too difficult, was what happened on the Sunday morning. Mrs B had hand-delivered the text of a dream from the previous night, in which the despairing child 'was crawling towards a motionless figure with the excited expectation of reaching this figure' (see Appendix, p. 132).

Two things in particular worried me about this communication. First, that I was being represented as 'motionless'. This reminded me of the long time in this analysis during which I had been held in place by the patient's defensive need to control me. This now felt like a warning, that Mrs B might be slipping back into a position in which I was barely allowed to function as analyst, as a person separate from herself.

I could argue that Mrs B might have needed to return to such a defensive position, and I would probably have been comfortable with that possibility were it not for the further fact of her feeling she had to bring this dream to me on the Sunday, rather than wait until her Monday session. Her not waiting to tell me this dream made me realize she was almost certainly feeling *I* might need to be reassured (and this was confirmed in the Monday session). It looked as if, in her mind, I might really not survive the weight of anxiety left with me on the Friday unless she helped me through the weekend by telling me *straight away* that she was feeling able to go on.

This rang many warning bells for me. This was in the area of Mrs B's belief that she would undoubtedly become too much for me. But *what* might be too much for me? Letting her hold my hand did not seem to be a problem to *me*. But she seemed already to be wondering why I had agreed to let her hold my hand. She also seemed (unconsciously) to intuit that the safer course *for me* would be with the possibility of her holding my hand still in place. I could then have counted on being able to return to a position of just listening to her narrative, rather than being more fully there for her as the object of her anxiety and rage.

My agreeing to Mrs B holding my hand had actually come from a failure of my courage. I did not see this as a failure of my abstinence but a failure to dare staying with the drift of my patient's material, all of her unconscious communication having so consistently pointed to her greatest fear. And that had not been a fear of remembering (she had long been remembering) but the fear of being too much for her mother, or for the 'other'.

Some discussants have assumed that I was afraid of physical contact with my patient, even of this token kind, and Breckenridge believes that my patient could see that I was afraid. However, the real fear that my patient sensed in me was not in the idea of her holding my hand but in what I would have to face if I were to *withdraw* that offer of my hand. And so it proved to be.

Breckenridge (2000: 8–9) goes on to say: 'the weekend seems to have convinced [Casement] that he wasn't afraid'. I have to disagree with this. It had in fact convinced me that I was much more afraid of what lay ahead in the analysis (as illustrated in the way it went), and I knew that I owed it to my patient to find sufficient courage for me to be able to overcome that fear – my *own* fear.

I had unconsciously registered that, in agreeing to an unusual exception to the boundaries of an analysis, I was almost certainly seeking to bypass something much more difficult that was around the corner. And we could still have avoided that if I had not rethought the hand-holding. But then the idea of withdrawing the possibility of Mrs B holding my hand seemed more than I could tolerate, despite this already being indicated through her seeing me as not surviving the pressures of the Friday session without her help.

Even though I had always been advocating the importance of continuing to follow the patient's communications, including the patient's unconscious prompts, here it seemed that Mrs B was drawing me towards something that was more than I could contemplate alone, especially if that might mean having to withdraw from her the possibility of holding my hand. I therefore sought an urgent consultation. I rang up the late Dr Paula Heimann who was already familiar with my work with Mrs B. She agreed to see me straight away – on the Sunday.

Dr Heimann confirmed my sense that I would be avoiding what seemed to be the worst thing in my patient's experience: the intensity of her feelings, assumed to be unmanageable. And it had already been evident that Mrs B had formed this view of her intense feelings, as too much for the 'other', in relation to her mother who had been unable to stay with her throughout the operation. If I were still to allow the possibility of Mrs B holding my hand, presenting myself as the 'better mother' still holding her hand through her reliving of that time in the transference, I would almost certainly be experienced by her as being either unwilling or unable to bear the impact of her distress. This had originally been directed at her mother who had fainted, apparently *because* of it. So, if I continued to behave as if I too had to avoid the intensity of her distress, this would undoubtedly have confirmed her deep conviction – that no one would be able to bear remaining in touch with her neediness, and her most intense feelings. Dr Heimann was therefore of the opinion that my avoidance here would almost certainly come to promote a similar avoidance in my patient, and that this could develop into a continuing avoidance of any really intense dependence upon anyone.

Although I was able to recognize what Dr Heimann was saying, I left the consultation still feeling I could not possibly withdraw my offer merely because this consultant was so sure that I should. In fact, I had said to Dr Heimann that I saw *no way* in which I could withdraw my agreement for Mrs B to hold my hand if it ever again became so difficult to bear. However, Dr Heimann had replied: 'Of course you must not introduce this from outside of your work with the patient. You can't do that just because *I* say so. The patient will lead you. *She will show you the way.*'

I felt fairly happy with this, as I had always believed in that approach. But on this occasion I was actually wishing to believe my patient would begin to lead me in some other direction. However, to my horror, in the very next session Mrs B began to see me as the figure she might reach, but *who was then seen as collapsing.* This was not just the first unconscious prompt from my patient that the hand-holding was not being as helpful as it was meant to be. Over the weekend, and in the first session after it, Mrs B was already seeing me as confirming her long-held belief that *no one* would be able to survive the impact of her most intense feelings. I had to take this in, and it is central to what I regard as 'learning from the patient' that we be prepared to learn even what we least want to know. And this was precisely what I least wanted to be hearing from my patient at that moment.

What about my countertransference during this time? I regret not having included more of my own exploring of this countertransference in the original paper (1982), as some of the misunderstandings that have emerged in subsequent discussions might have been avoided.

On the Friday I had been trying to explore (prematurely as it turned out) what may have been around for Mrs B in the time before the accident. I had been wanting to believe we had already negotiated the worst of this patient's traumatic childhood, in her re-experiencing of the accident,[5] not wanting to consider that there could be something worse still to come: worse also for me. At this moment, therefore, I was the one who was defensively taking flight to the past. My countertransference was picking up something of what else might lie ahead. And I now know that I had been defensively deflecting the patient, and myself, from whatever that might be. My unconscious manoeuvre, in effect, had been aimed at keeping the worst of that experience (her not being held and her response to it) still outside the session. Then, with the help of my patient's prompts, I could no longer avoid seeing the more crucial issue for her: that her analyst was being experienced as 'collapsing'.

It was only much later in this analysis that Mrs B learned from her mother a quite new fact: that the only hospital she could have been taken to (after the burning) was known then to be in no fit state to care for a patient with such severe burns. The doctor thought the baby would die if she were to be sent to that hospital, and there were reasons why she could not be taken to any other. Consequently, the best chance of her surviving would be if her mother could nurse her at home. But that would mean 'barrier nursing', i.e. *not holding her or touching her* except with sterilized gloves, and then only for the most minimal and essential feeding and cleaning. Whatever she did, the mother must not pick up her baby, however much she cried for this. For, if the mother did pick her up it might

5 This has previously been described in detail in Chapter 5 of *On Learning from the Patient* (1985) and Chapter 5 of *Learning from the Patient* (1991).

lead to her baby dying from infection, and there was no antibiotic treatment available at that time. What a parallel! So, we can imagine the agonies her mother must have gone through as she cared for her, whilst having to inhibit the natural impulse of a mother to hold her distressed baby to herself, to give her the hugs that are meant to 'make it better'.

Strangely, I had gone through similar agonies in my countertransference, in being there for my patient's distress, wishing so strongly that my patient could at least have had the reassurance of my hand to help her through that experience.

At the time, what I was doing in not holding her hand made no more sense to Mrs B (consciously) than it did to those discussants who have disagreed with my handling of this case. And yet, the main thing that got me through that awful time (and it was many months before it began to feel in any sense better) was my becoming aware of my patient's unconscious communications. It was through these that I had been prompted to see the implications of my choice, and to see what was required of me at this point in the analysis.

From my own previous work with Mrs B I had come to realize she was unconsciously convinced that no one, just *no one*, would be able to survive being in the presence of her rage, her neediness and her despair: *all* that seemed to have caused her mother to collapse. And Mrs B's alarm had been related to her thought that I too seemed to be collapsing.

The issue of my surviving the intensity of her feelings had therefore emerged as central. I had been seeing only some of it at first, but fortunately seeing enough to sense that I had to find the courage to go through this with Mrs B, and not to bypass it.

As I have said, I needed a quite new courage to grasp the nettle, and to be 'there' for Mrs B throughout many months while she felt sure I had acted out of cowardice, and while she raged at me for this. It was only by following my patient through each and every session that I could find a way through. None of this could have been negotiated by rule, even less by rule alone.

I could not have stood by my decision (to withdraw the offer of my hand) had it been made simply on the basis of a rule; nor indeed if it had been merely upon the advice of a consultant, however much I respected her. It was in my patient's own communications, both in the present sequence and in the wider context of the analysis as a whole, that I was being so clearly prompted to act as I did. And I was being prompted at a level which was far more significant than any of the surface communication.

I do not regret having followed my patient as I did, though there were many occasions during this when I wondered if I had been mistaken.

Frequently I *wanted* to believe I could have been mistaken. That would have allowed me, after all, to capitulate to the pressures from my patient as she consciously so wished that I would.

My patient too does not regret that I stayed with my decision to follow her prompts. It was not a matter of 'persuading' her to agree with me, as has been suggested. Mrs B, at the very end of her analysis, selected this sequence in particular as the time that had been most central in her analysis and most crucial to her. This had finally given her a chance to *refind the mother who had helped to save her life*: strangely re-found through my *not* holding her.

Until then, Mrs B had always thought of her mother as having been cruel to her, in not being there when she had most needed her, particularly at the time of the accident and subsequently with the surgeon. Her mother, she only later discovered, had in fact managed to be 'there' for her *in the barrier nursing* (at that earlier time) despite the appearance of not being. And, it should be noted, the loss of her mother's hand, at the time of the operation, was all the more traumatic for Mrs B because (unknown to her or to me) this so exactly repeated the absence of her mother's hands throughout that period of barrier nursing. But we did not know this at the time.

It seems now that there had been a most extraordinary 'parallel process' around when I learned of the mother's contribution to her baby's recovery from the burns, *in not holding* her, so uncannily replicated in my own not holding of Mrs B during this time in her analysis. Also, her mother could not have managed this alone. She had a doctor behind her, telling her how important it was that she nurse her baby without doing that most natural thing a mother would want to do under the circumstances. And I, similarly, could not have found the courage to go through this period in the analysis, without that holding, had I not also had a doctor helping me not to swerve from following my patient's unconscious communication. That was really what I had to follow throughout: by no means just following a rule of abstinence.

So this is what I mean by learning from the patient. It was not a matter of just following the rules that classical analysts have chosen to follow. It meant following the patient and daring to go where the patient unconsciously prompted me to go. My struggle was not 'how to stay true to the rule' but 'how to remain true to my patient'.

Chapter 8

Impingement and space: issues of technique

When travelling in unknown territory it helps to have some landmarks, or some identifiable stars, by which one can find one's bearings.

In relation to psychoanalytic technique, I think of impingement[1] and space as two sides of a coin. To be protected from impingement we need space. However, the analytic space and process can so easily be disturbed by impingements.

Winnicott was acutely sensitive to the impact of impingements and the ways in which these can affect development in an infant.

> In the early development of the human being the environment that behaves well enough (that makes good enough active adaptation) enables personal growth to take place. If the environment behaves not well enough, then the individual is engaged in reactions to impingement, and the self processes are interrupted.
>
> From this one can formulate a fundamental principle of existence: that which proceeds from the true self feels real (later good) whatever its nature, however aggressive; that which happens in the individual as a reaction to environmental impingement feels unreal, futile (later bad), however sensually satisfactory.
>
> (Winnicott, 1955: 25)

Winnicott recognized this principle in relation to infants, but it also has far-reaching implications for psychoanalytic technique.

---

1 Winnicott defined impingement, in relation to an infant, as 'something that interrupts the continuity of being' (Winnicott, 1956).

Winnicott was emphatic about the importance for an infant, even from birth, to be able to resist what is presented to it by the mother or other carer. Without that freedom to reject, to say 'No', the infant remains helplessly vulnerable to whatever is presented, the manner and timing otherwise being totally outside of its control. Even though patients are not helpless in exactly that way, the analytic experience can also be profoundly affected by impingements from the analyst.

Some analysts seem to see themselves as there to control the analysis. But there is an important difference between an analyst there to contain, and in that sense to be in control, and an analyst dominating the process. Much depends upon whose initiative determines what comes into any given session, not only at the start (in terms of how a session begins[2]) but from moment to moment throughout a session.

Through being alert to impingements we may find a useful guide on issues of technique. For instance, it can help us to be alert to the way in which we are speaking to patients, and treating them, and possibly impinging upon them in ways that could have far-reaching effects upon how an analysis develops.

As mentioned in Chapter 1, an analysis will develop in quite different ways depending upon how closely the analyst stays with and respects what a patient is bringing to the current session. When the analyst brings in something (however relevant it may seem to be) from a previous session, much will depend upon how closely this relates to what the patient has been speaking of so far. The analyst may see some connection. But if the patient doesn't see this, the new matter that is brought in by the analyst (rather than by the patient) is likely to be experienced as belonging to the analyst's agenda, not the patient's. Something introduced by the analyst can then highjack a session, deflecting it from where it might otherwise have gone had the direction been more clearly determined by the patient. It can also shift the initiative for a session away from the patient to the analyst. And if the patient too often goes along with this it can lead the patient into compliance, and into a compliant relationship to the analyst.

Compliance, as Winnicott often pointed out, contributes to false-self development. By contrast, it is usually assumed that psychoanalysis is

---

2 It is not only through speech that patients start a session. I therefore do not think that we always have to wait for a patient to speak first, as if this were some kind of ritual of analysis. Instead, it is sometimes appropriate to respond to the quality of an initial silence, taking this also as a communication that can at least be acknowledged.

concerned with what is true and genuine for the patient. But sometimes patients find themselves in an analysis in which they feel dominated and controlled by the analyst.

The analyst's sensitivity to impingement can therefore provide a useful touchstone by which we can test our technique in analysis. Are we truly following a patient or are we leading? Are we really being responsive to the patient's communications or are we making declarations about the patient's unconscious on the basis of theory? Are we following the patient's unconscious prompts and cues, by which we can be helped to reorientate our thinking when necessary, or are we ignoring these or not seeing them? Are we staying long enough with an honest not-knowing, while we wait to hear more from the patient, or are we tending to select only those bits of what we hear from a patient that fit in with our own preconceptions and what our theory may lead us to expect? Do our attempts to interpret come across to the patient as motivated by a concern to understand? Or, may some interpretations be experienced as criticism, as complaint, as an attempt to demonstrate who is in control, or whatever else? And when patients indicate that they are experiencing the analyst in such ways as these, are we prepared to accept that this may be in response to how we have actually been addressing them? Do we then try to rectify our technique, or do we continue to see what is happening in terms of the patient's pathology rather than as something to be considered interactionally, as co-created?[3]

Analysts can impinge upon their patients in countless ways, and it is rather surprising that this dimension to the analytic process seems to be so often overlooked. It raises important questions about the nature of the analytic endeavour. Some patients, finding themselves with one kind of analyst, feel that they discover a freedom in which they can begin to become more fully themselves. Others, with another kind of analyst, seem

---

3 Arlene Kramer Richards, reporting on Philip Bromberg's contribution to discussion, writes: 'Within an interpersonal-relational model, the transferential intensity that leads to genuine analytic experience is co-created through the real, not "implied," interaction between the participants, and it is the analyst's ability to observe his or her contribution to an enactment that is the critical element in enabling patients to see themselves through the analyst's eyes and make use of interpretations (1997: 1241). Another view on this may be found in a report on a meeting of the Psychoanalytic Association of New York, in which Steven Snyder writes: 'However, Dr. Blum took issue with those who would conclude from this that transference is "co-created" or is an interpersonal phenomenon. The transference is still the patient's creation, although obviously influenced in complex ways by reality' (1993: 704).

to experience pressures to see things as the analyst sees them, and feel dominated by the authority of the analyst. There is potentially such an inequality in psychoanalysis that it can result in a kind of relationship which, in any other sphere, might be regarded as unhealthy, even as sado-masochistic, with one party claiming rights over the other which cannot effectively be challenged.

It is worrying to hear sometimes of patients who are apparently 'having a terrible time with their analyst', where the relationship described seems to be one in which the patient feels dominated, even crushed, by the analyst's authority over all matters of the unconscious. Of course it cannot be assumed that any such account by a discontented patient is necessarily objective. Nevertheless, we do sometimes hear of analysts who seem to see all their patients predominantly in negative terms: as destructive, envious, greedy, manipulative, devious, grandiose, narcissistic, arrogant, contemptuous of the analyst, and much else.

Some patients *can* be like this. And when they are we have to be prepared to engage vigorously with such issues as these, otherwise we will be experienced as avoiding them. But it does not have to be that all patients are necessarily as full of destructiveness as some analysts seem to assume. Therefore, if an analyst sees a patient almost exclusively in such negative terms it may be because there is a battle for control which does not have to be all caused by the patient.

Some children are treated in these ways, parents seeing them almost exclusively as bad. It is not surprising that we quite often find such children later developing a distorted view of themselves, even seeing themselves as capable of little other than being bad. So how is it that an analyst can impact upon a patient in such similar ways to these, without seeming to be concerned about how this may impinge upon the analytic relationship?

Among the justifications put forward for treating patients in these harrying ways is the notion that the bad in the patient would otherwise dominate the analysis, or that the destructiveness in the patient would never be properly exposed or analysed. But it has been my experience that the difficult aspects of a patient can be dealt with very differently, provided that a patient is given the opportunity to feel safe enough within the analytic relationship for these to be brought into the analysis more spontaneously. There can be plenty of opportunity to engage with the destructive side of patients without provoking the very thing we are trying to analyse.

There are times (as also noted in Chapter 2) when we find that a patient is being arrogant, or narcissistic, or whatever. We are then faced with a choice as to whether we approach this in a way that can sound critical or in a way that indicates our attempts at understanding. What can help us then is to recover our analytic curiosity. And I have always valued hearing Bion speak of a time when he found himself falling into a state of extreme boredom with a patient. Then, just before succumbing to this into sleep, he was able to recover what he called his 'analytic curiosity'. Stimulated by this, he was able to wonder how could anyone be so boring? He was then no longer bored because he now had this fascinating question to consider. Likewise, we can wonder about what lies beneath any behaviour or attitude in patients that we might otherwise be inclined to criticize.

Monitoring for our own (potentially) pathogenic impingements upon patients can often help us to clean up our technique so that we do not unnecessarily muddy the very waters that we are trying to clarify.[4] Our being aware of the use of analytic space can similarly help us to monitor our work with a patient.

What do I mean by 'space'?

Space in analysis, in the more general sense, may be thought of as the interpersonal space between the patient and the analyst, which we try as far as possible to keep free from intrusion, interference or influence, whether from outside the analysis or from the analyst. Whatever happens within this space is normally all part of the analysis.

However, the analytic space is much more than just the setting within which an analysis takes place, with its professional framework and the necessary boundaries of privacy and confidentiality. It is also the emotional space between the analyst and the patient, a space that may be bridged by the patient reaching out to the analyst or by the analyst reaching out to the patient. It may be filled, in one way or another, or be left empty: a space for thinking, a space for relating, a space for experiencing and for being. The initiative for the use of this space is usually left to the patient.[5]

The notion of analytic space (as with impingement) may therefore help as a context for monitoring what is happening between the analyst and the patient: how this space is being used and by whom. When it is the analyst who 'puts' something into the analytic space, the patient is usually very sensitive to this and to what it may indicate about the analyst, as that

4 See 'The persecutory therapist' (Meares and Hobson, 1977); also 'On Iatrogenia' (Marrone, 1998: Chapter 12).
5 Britton (1998) uses the notion of space in quite different and interesting ways, speaking of *triangular space* and *poetic space*.

may also have implications for the patient.[6] Unconsciously, a patient will always notice who puts what into this space.

Further, if it is going to be possible for the transference to be analysed, there has to be a *sufficient difference* between the objective realities in an analysis and whatever is being transferred. The patient has to be able to distinguish one from the other. Without this sufficient difference the analyst is likely to be experienced as being too much the same as some object relationship in the past, which may preclude any attempt at analysing this with the patient. Jay Greenberg, in his paper 'On the analyst's neutrality', says of this: 'If the analyst cannot be experienced as a new object, analysis never gets under way; if he cannot be experienced as an old one, it never ends' (1986: 98).

In a more crucial sense, the analytic space represents a freedom to do convincing analytic work on what is happening within the analytic relationship: either a mental space within which the patient can move between what the analyst interprets and what the patient makes of that interpretation, or the space between the realities of the analytic relationship and the transference. If an interpretation leaves no room for the patient, except to agree or disagree, the patient has no space for his/her own thinking. And if the objective realities of the analytic relationship are too similar to the transference the patient will not be able to distinguish one from the other; then the analytic work may become impossible and result in impasse.

Example

> I once heard an analyst boasting of how he had apparently 'cured' an attractive female patient from going to sleep in her sessions with him. He had been reflecting upon the phenomenon of her sleeping in his presence and he had imagined that it represented an unacknowledged wish. He had therefore interpreted this to the patient as her wish to *sleep with him*. The patient became immediately alert and she never slept in a session again!

---

6 An important exception to this is when there is something important being avoided from an earlier session. (A glaring example of this can be found in Chapter 6 when I failed to comment on my patient making no reference to my repeated mistakes.) I think that it is then useful to wait until the avoidance is sufficiently evident for the patient to be able to recognize this when attention is drawn to it. There is often something of value to learn from the avoidance too.

If we trial-identify with the patient here, we can wonder how this patient may have heard this interpretation – particularly as it might have revealed what had been in her analyst's mind more clearly than anything that had been in her own. She could therefore have heard this as evidence that *he* had thoughts about sleeping with *her*, in which case the change in her behaviour might not have expressed the accuracy of his interpretation (as the analyst had assumed) so much as her alarm at being alone in a room, lying on a couch in the presence of an analyst who had, in effect, admitted to having such thoughts about her.

I think it is likely that the analytic space, for this patient, could no longer be regarded as a safe place in which she could relax without feeling a need to be on guard against the possibility of her analyst having sexual thoughts about her. The analytic space would then have become constricted.

Example

A homosexual patient had come for an initial consultation with me and I had agreed to take him into analysis. At the end of this consultation he asked me about parking his scooter when he came for his sessions. He had noticed a scooter already parked alongside the path leading to my front door. Could he put his scooter there too when he came for his sessions?[7] I now think of this question as a 'banana skin', a question that has a hidden agenda which is asked when there is no time to consider what the implications might be in trying to answer it.

I was very inexperienced then, this being the second supervised case in my psychoanalytic training, and I failed to recognize that this question might well be a complicated enquiry. I now know that it would have been better to have left this unanswered until we had discovered more of what was being communicated by my patient through his enquiry. For instance, I might have said something like: 'I don't feel able to answer your question just now as I am not yet clear what you might be *telling* me in asking it. But we can return to this, if you wish, in the course of your analysis.' It could then have been left for the patient to bring up again at some later time – if he wished. Unfortunately, I answered his question at the level of

---

7   This was many years ago, at a time when there was no problem in parking on the road outside of my house.

objective reality, saying: 'I don't think you will find that there is room for two scooters there.'

This patient subsequently revealed that he had interpreted my response as indicating that I was afraid of his homosexuality, and I have to acknowledge that (in those days) there may have been some truth in this. I had not previously worked with a homosexual patient, and this patient immediately sensed the unconscious communication from me in my reply. My countertransference here may therefore have been on the side of keeping this patient, to begin with, at a distance. But it would have made for a less clumsy start to this analysis if I had recognized this caution in myself, and dealt with it differently through being more alert to the implications in the patient's question. As it was, we had to do the initial work of this analysis while the patient was convinced that I was afraid of letting him get close to me, as an objective reality (partly confirmed by me) rather than as a manifestation of his transference. I had unwittingly blurred the distinction between these two realities, and it took a long time to recover a more neutral, and essential, space for the analysis in relation to this issue.

There also needs to be a space between how the patient sees something and how the analyst speaks of it. For instance, I was pleased to hear a supervisee respond carefully to her patient with this is mind (see following example).

Example

PATIENT: I think you disapprove of my negative feelings.
THERAPIST: We need to understand better your own idea of what you regard as 'negative feelings'.

This is an example of where it would have been a mistake merely to use the patient's own language, without some challenging of it. The therapeutic task here needs to be in the area of questioning the patient's view of his feelings as negative, which might then throw light on why he expects disapproval. It would have been much harder to explore that if the therapist's own language had already been that of disapproval.

The notion of space in an analysis can help us to recognize our own contributions to the ebb and flow of the analytic process. I find the notion of space, in this respect, more useful than Freud's idea of the analyst as a blank screen. The ideal of the blank screen is less dynamic: it states how things should be in an analysis, rather than how things are. By contrast, the notion of space can prompt us to recognize what is happening between the patient and the analyst. It is not just a matter of what is being projected, or transferred, onto the analyst.

Space and theories of technique

A key difference between those analysts who have little use for the notion of space, and those who believe it has an important function in analysis, is I believe largely due to different theoretical views with regard to pathology and the related theories of the analytic process and processes of cure.

Some analysts see pathology as stemming primarily from destructive forces within the personality. They are then likely to take less account of the impact of environmental failure (Winnicott, 1955), concentrating instead upon the ways in which even the earliest object relationships may have been disturbed by destructive forces such as the death instinct and innate envy.[8] And when the preferred theory happens to see pathology as more due to innate destructiveness than to environmental influence, the analytic process can become dominated by a pursuit of anything seen as 'bad' in a patient, insufficient regard being shown for the patient's history. (At least this is how some patients have described their experience of a previous analysis.) Neglect of the realities of what may actually have happened in a patient's childhood, when the analytic focus is predominantly on the 'here and now', seems often to be parallelled by a comparable neglect of the realities within the analytic relationship and of the analyst's ways of working.

Unfortunately, the disturbing effects of the analyst's style of clinical work can be much more easily overlooked when there is to hand a theory of explanation that can attribute all disturbance[9] in an analysis to the pathology of the patient. With a view of disturbance as predominantly

---

8 It concerns me greatly that some analysts use the notion of 'envy of the good breast' as a way of fending off criticism that might otherwise be valid and helpful. Melanie Klein, who coined this notion, seemed to attribute difficulties with her own children to this envy of her as a good mother. What can then be left out here is the extent to which children have been responding to the way they were *actually* mothered.

9 What I mean by 'disturbance' here is anything from the analyst that either disturbs the natural flow of the analytic process, such as deflecting this or directing it along lines selected by the analyst, or anything that brings about the appearance of psychological disturbance in the patient. This may become evident in response to the analyst's treatment of the patient rather than being a true expression of the patient's own state of mind.

internal to the patient, it may seem that there is not much need for this analytic space, within which to consider what also happens between the analyst and the patient. I have even heard it argued that it might be colluding with a patient's resistance to *allow* space to the patient, as if the aim of analysis were to track down and to eliminate 'bad' in the patient rather than to provide a sufficient sense of safety within the analytic relationship for the patient to dare to be less defended.

In contrast to the above, there are other analysts (like Winnicott) who consider the caregiving function of the mother or mother-person to be supremely important. They trace the effects of environmental influence from birth, if not from before. They are careful to take into account these external realities of the childhood history and, by logical extension, the external reality of the analytic relationship – however much this may also be distorted by the patient's projections and transference(s), which are known to affect all relating.

Space for playing and space for being

Another function of analytic space is for playing and for being. To that end, we can profitably consider what Winnicott has said of the processes between a mother and her baby in which playing becomes possible. In *Playing and Reality*, Winnicott writes: 'The mother (or part of mother) is in a "to and fro" between being that which the baby has a capacity to find and (alternatively) being herself waiting to be found' (1971b: 47). I take this to mean that there is so much more of the mother to be found, that the baby is not yet ready for, which the mother keeps in abeyance for when her baby *is* ready for this.

It is the mother's willingness to be reliably but non-intrusively present for her baby that becomes the basis for her baby's capacity to play. The baby can then use the mother either as present or as absent, and yet (paradoxically) it is only because her background presence is being taken for granted that this playing is possible. With the older child (which can also apply to patients) it is the mother's return from a temporary absence that is relied upon that enables a child to play creatively rather than obsessively, even when alone.

Patients in analysis can arrive at a similar use of the analyst for creative play, which for some patients can be the very essence of psychoanalysis. But only under certain conditions. If an analyst too often gives his interpretations as unquestionable fact, the patient is left with little more than the two options of accepting or challenging. There is then no room for playing with an idea, the patient kicking it around whilst offering other angles that could also be considered. By contrast, there will usually be more space for the patient to play with interpretations when these are presented in a tentative form, or when the analyst shares his own not-knowing as well as what he believes he is beginning to understand. Dogmatic interpreting, on the other hand, can too easily create an atmosphere of battle, which is not necessarily a phenomenon of transference nor is it an inevitable feature of the analytic process. And in battle there is usually little space for freedom of thought or for being.

Analytic space in relation to interpretations

It is always important that we leave room for a patient to do something with an interpretation beyond just agreeing with it or disagreeing.

Example

> In supervision I heard a student therapist report having said to his female patient: 'You are guilty about having wished your brother dead.' This was said in the context of the patient's brother having recently died, and I could recognize the student's wish to open up the issue of the patient's guilt-reactions to this death. But the patient could hear this quite differently from how it was intended.

The confrontation, put in this way, could feel as if the therapist has sided with the patient's superego, apparently accusing her of having wished her brother dead – perhaps even accusing her of having caused it. If we trial-identify with the patient here we can readily sense how she could feel cornered by this. What could she do with it? She could perhaps say: 'Yes, I am guilty of that.' Or she might defend herself from this statement, as from an accusation.

The point that the therapist is trying to get to is, of course, that the patient (as a child) may have wished this, and may be accusing herself on account of it. So, in order to preserve the analytic space and the possibility of questioning the unconscious links in the patient's mind (rather than seeming to reinforce them) therapists have to be careful to leave room for more than one view on what they are trying to examine with a patient.

It would have been preferable, therefore, if the therapist had said something like: 'We still need to understand why you feel guilty about your brother's death.' At least the therapist would not sound as if he thought the patient *should* feel guilty. The patient might then recall her own resentment at her brother's birth, as if her early wish to have her brother out of the way might now explain her sense of guilt. This could have opened up an enquiry into the assumptions of magical thinking, the patient feeling as if the wishes of childhood had the power to bring about a fulfilment of those wishes. The space, which is essential here for a more open-ended exploration of this issue, would then have been better preserved. That would have left room for the patient also *not* to feel guilty. By contrast, when a superego attitude is emanating from the analyst, this can seriously restrict the analytic space. The patient can then feel as if that is what he/she *should* feel.

An extended example

> Mr A, who had for some time been seriously suicidal, had recently been feeling slightly better. He then brought a dream fragment in which *he had been filling up his car with petrol. The strange thing about this was that the petrol pump was by a hedge that was in front of a private house.* He had no further thoughts.

Internal supervision

This (female) analyst's associations in the session were to a journey, wanting to believe that Mr A might be feeling ready to move on from his suicidal brooding to continue his life's journey. However, she also remembered that, when he had previously been most persistently suicidal, he had planned to kill himself with exhaust fumes from his car. He had bought some rubber piping for that purpose, and he still had it. The analyst then did not know whether this dream indicated a move on from his acute depression; or, possibly, it might indicate a return to the idea of suicidal action. She therefore felt she had to be careful not to make any interpretation that might exclude the continuing risk of suicide, even though it was tempting to think of this dream as suggesting some preparation for a journey.

The analyst also noticed that, in this dream, there might be a reference to the hedge in front of her house (also a private house), which Mr A passed each time he came to his analysis.

Comment

The analyst could have waited for the patient to speak, to give his own associations to his dream, and some might suggest that she should have waited.

> Mr A continued to be silent, so (after a pause) the analyst added: 'There is a hedge in front of *my* house.'

Comment

In supervision, the analyst said that she had offered this observation as a way of inviting the patient to return to speaking, and maybe to give his own further thoughts about the dream.

> Mr A replied: 'Oh, yes, so there is.' As he was then again silent for quite some time, the analyst continued: 'If this dream refers to your coming here, I think it may indicate that you are still looking to me to fill up the emptiness within you.'

Comment

In supervision, the analyst explained that she was being careful not to assume that the patient experiences her as *actually* filling that emptiness.

> Mr A replied: 'Yes, but I still do not know where my journey might be going.'

Discussion

What the analyst has tried to do here is to keep the analytic space open for all possibilities, not to foreclose on any of the potential meanings in the dream. So far Mr A seems to be doing the same.

The options that remain open for further exploration include the possibility that the patient may or may not be finding what he needs from the analyst. Also, he may or may not use the petrol in his dream to continue with his life's journey, or he might still be wondering whether to use this in the service of his own death. And, in his reply, he acknowledges that he still does not know where he is going. However, it is to be hoped that he can sense the analyst is open to these very different possibilities.

If, instead, the analyst had suggested that she was being dreamed of as *providing* him with what he needed to continue his journey, the patient could have heard her as out of touch with his continuing thoughts of suicide. The analytic space in that case would have been seriously limited, as the patient would have had to contend with the analyst's intrusive and deflective wish to see him getting on with his life, as if she could not tolerate the possibility that he might still be contemplating suicide. And, had she come across to him as being out of touch with this, he could have experienced her as unbearably too much like others in his life who had not remained in touch with what he was feeling, particularly when he could not bear that alone.

If we are to maximize our chance of following where the patient is going, of his/her own accord and uninfluenced by us, it is important that we keep the analytic space as free as we can from any avoidable input from ourselves that could prompt the patient to follow a direction that is being determined by us and not by the patient.

Impingement and space in relation to technique

As I have tried to illustrate, it is always useful to consider our own contribution to a session in relation to both impingement and space. How are we being in the session? What are we bringing to the session, and why? Does it belong in this session? Is it truly in response to what the patient has been bringing to this session, or are we deflecting from this by bringing in something from elsewhere? Are we *finding* connections that are dynamically present in the patient's overall communication, or are we merely *making* connections? Also, in terms of the quality of our interventions, are these neutral or are they in some way loaded?

The nature of the analytic relationship is determined by many such issues as these. And it is only when the analytic space is sufficiently free for the patient's own personal use that we can engage with what truly comes from within the patient's own mind, rather than putting our ideas (and our theory) *into* the mind of the patient. Quite different kinds of analysis are likely to follow from the different ways in which we approach these issues, seeing them as central or seeing them as only peripheral. The difference for patients can be between the analytic opportunity to become more fully themselves or becoming in some way moulded into a version of the analyst. And at the end of an analysis, to what extent are patients identified with the analyst ('a chip off the old block') and to what extent have they grown more fully into the people that they have the potential to become?

Chapter 9

The unknown beyond the known[1]

A sure way of getting lost is to rely upon a familiar map in unfamiliar territory.

Introduction

This chapter aims to address some of the errors that we can make in mistaking the unknown for what is already more familiar, and the value in waiting until we are able to see beyond this.

First, I wish to consider some of the processes by which we relate to each other, in particular to somebody not yet known to us, and some of the obstacles that can get in the way of *really* knowing them. These processes are around in all of life no less than in the analytic encounter. To begin with, therefore, I shall be considering them in ordinary and familiar settings, but it will become apparent that these descriptions are offered as metaphors for aspects of the analytic encounter.

Meeting the unfamiliar

From birth we structure our experience, linking like with like. The unfamiliar is examined in its strangeness until some sense of it can be attained. Or it is turned away from as uninteresting or as threatening, as there can sometimes be a deep disquiet when we are faced by something that is unfamiliar.

---

1 This chapter was first presented at an Independent Group Conference 'Getting to know somebody new', held at University College, London, in November 1994.

At first, as an infant, we have limited structures to relate to. However, as our experience widens so does our repertoire of what can be referred to in assessing somebody new. Much then depends upon our interest in meeting somebody we hardly know, as to how much we feel we need to ascertain before we can begin to think that we know them.

An example from everyday life

When two people meet for the first time, there are customary rituals by which they seek to lessen the unease that is inherent in meeting someone unknown. At a party, for example, the things that are commonly said include such questions as: 'What do you do?' or 'Do you live around here?' Then, from enquiries like these, it is usually possible to place the other person sufficiently to begin to feel that some *common ground* has been found. Or, failing that, at least some way of locating the other may have been achieved.

Stereotypes

There can be no genuine short-cuts towards deeply knowing another person. It could take a lifetime. Even if we live intimately with another person, can we ever say we really know them? But we are always taking short-cuts, and one of the most common is that of stereotyping.

For instance, when we meet strangers, once we have learned something like what job they do, we are already entering the process of building up a picture of them. We may then begin to think we can put them into a familiar category. From our previous knowledge of people in that category we may begin think that we know more about them than we really do. But gaining a proper sense of what is most important, and individual, about a stranger will take much fuller exploration. However, when we are impatient to remove a sense of strangeness, and the unease of not-knowing, we sometimes settle for what is familiar. We can see this happening in some clinical work too.

Relating to the unfamiliar

When we do not find common ground with a stranger we will often draw upon our experience of other people. But there are dangers here, because we tend to limit our openness to what is not known by obscuring this with whatever seems familiar. We may thus transfer onto the unfamiliar from other relationships, treating something about this new person as if he/she were more like someone else than might be the case. Or we may project from ourselves, in ways that will blur the distinctions between familiar and unfamiliar, by treating these differences as secondary. But so often it is with these differences in particular that we should be most concerned, for it is here especially that we will encounter what is most individual and unique about the other.

There is more than one interesting divide here. As with the optimist, who sees the same glass of water as the pessimist, but who regards it as half full rather than half empty, so with the familiar and the unfamiliar. There are those who tend to be too confident, thinking they already know the other (even on limited evidence), and there are those who may feel paralysed from making any generalization on the grounds that they feel they always need to know more. And amongst the too confident are those who can become arrogant in their belief that they are expert in knowing about people. But there are also those who may become suspicious, even paranoid, in their ill-founded certainties about the other. Each in their own ways, and for quite different reasons, places the other in whatever categories are assumed to fit. However, assumptions and preconception are always inimical to knowing the other more genuinely.

The contribution of theory and of other clinical experience

There are quite a few parallels between the task of an analyst trying to know a patient and a mother getting to know her baby. In each, there is usually some turning to book knowledge as well as drawing upon other experience.

With a first baby, a mother is often anxious and likely to consult books or to seek advice from others with more experience of babies than she has. Armed then with that advice and with what she has gained from her observation of other mothers, and drawing upon her own (mostly unconscious) experience of having been a baby, she may feel able to approach the task of getting to know *her* newborn baby. But this guidance from others has the disadvantage of not being about her own baby. At best, as Winnicott often pointed out, it can only be about an average baby or about babies in general.

However, when a mother has found her feet with her first baby she may begin to feel that she now 'knows' about babies. So, with a subsequent baby some mothers overlook that they are again faced with someone entirely new. They may have learned how to 'read' a first baby, but a sensitive mother knows that she has to learn much of this again, learning afresh how to be the mother that each baby needs, at each stage of development.

Similarly, with a first patient, student analysts are naturally anxious and they are likely to draw quite heavily upon what has been learned from others, as from their own analyst or a supervisor. But, again, none of the guidance that can be gained from those sources will bear as directly upon the patient in question as might be wished. Student analysts therefore have much to learn from their patients, concerning how to relate *what they know* to *what they still do not know*, and how to become the analyst that each patient most needs to find at each stage of an analysis.

As with a mother and her growing child, the awareness of changing need is discovered by the analyst/therapist with regard to what fits and what does not fit. Therefore, if a student relies too much on other experience this can get in the way of recognizing the (unconscious) prompts and cues of the particular patient. It is by no means the case that the analyst, even an experienced analyst, always knows better than the patient.

Of course we cannot hope to be able to work only on the basis of experience – our own or that of others – in getting to know a patient. In addition we rely on theory. But the question then is *how much* do we rely on this? And what if the theory is mistaken or does not apply as universally as we might like to think? Also, how does a general theory relate to the individual patient?

All analysts need to draw upon theory to help understand the unknown that confronts them in their patients throughout each analysis. But it is likely that students and recently qualified analysts will find themselves depending more upon theory, as they do not yet have extensive clinical experience to draw on. Understandably, the maps provided by theory may seem like a godsend to an inexperienced analyst when confronted by a new patient, or by a patient who is beginning to lead the analyst into unfamiliar territory. The urge then is to limit this sense of strangeness, to make the unfamiliar *seem* more familiar. Sometimes, however, the result (for the analyst) is an illusion of familiarity, and of pseudo-understanding, that may give the analyst a sense of security but may not give the patient a secure sense of being understood.

In contrast to student analysts, who know that they have limited experience to draw on, trained analysts need to beware of times when they could become *too confident* in their understanding. The more clinical experience one has, the easier it is to feel that there is nothing much new to be discovered in the consulting room. But there are serious risks in this attitude. For the individual is always new, and the insight that can be most meaningful to patients themselves is usually that which is discovered afresh with each particular person.

The unknown of the other

In all that I have said so far I have been trying to show how most of our researches bring us back to the familiar, either to that which we know from our own personal experience, or to that which seems familiar because of other clinical experience or theory. But whatever is truly unknown to us will always lie beyond the familiar, and beyond what we expect to find.

Analysts are used to thinking about that which is *unknown to the patient*: unknown because unconscious. Therefore, as they listen to a patient's communications, they are noting in particular what may be derived from some unconscious phantasy or memory. And gradually they hope to be able to piece together a clearer sense of the patient's internal world, to be able to interpret the unconscious so that it can become conscious to the patient. This is the daily task of every analyst, with much of it being familiar. And through this analytic work patients may begin to recognize what they previously had not known about themselves.

But, beyond the well-trodden paths of analytic practice, there lies that which still remains *unknown to the analyst*, and which may require a fundamental change of perspective for the analyst to be able to comprehend. For example, a change of viewpoint is sometimes necessary when an analyst is not yet able to take on board a patient's quite different experience of life, perhaps different from anything yet encountered by the analyst. Or, it may be necessary because the analyst is being blocked by a theoretical view that focuses attention onto some preconception or preoccupation, leading *away* from the patient's actual experience or from the more immediate communication of the moment.

There are thus problems when an analyst is not sufficiently familiar with the world of a particular patient, whether external or internal.

Example

> I vividly recall a time when I had to set aside what I had previously thought of as 'a mother' in order to tune into the quite different experience a patient had of *her* mother.
>
> This patient thought I was being sadistic when I said she was look-ing to me 'for mothering'. By this I did not mean that I was offering to be in the role of a mother. But I had sensed that she needed me to be there for her distress, which I think of as an important function

of mothering. She had always been afraid to turn to another person for emotional help, and I sensed she needed to be able to turn to me for that. But what she heard, in what I said, was something entirely different.

This patient, I then learned, *had* sometimes taken her distress to her mother when she was very small. But she had then learned not to expect any help with it. Instead, she usually felt attacked for upsetting her mother.

For this patient, a mother was someone who must not be upset; she was someone who must not be turned to in distress, and she was someone who would not help to make her child feel better, but would most likely make her feel worse. It therefore took this patient a long time to arrive at a different view of what a mother could be and what mothering might mean.

What was familiar to that patient was not yet familiar to me. I could only learn of it from her. Neither my personal experience nor my previous clinical practice had led me to see the idea of mothering in the way that this patient saw it. If anything, my preconception had been that even a deprived and damaged patient would have a notion of mothering, as something she had needed even if she had been deprived of it. In fact, so afraid had this patient been of anything to do with mothers, she had been terrified of ever becoming a mother herself. So my world and hers (as regards mothers) had been completely different, and I had to find a bridge between these very different worlds. But first, I had to recognize the gulf between her experience and mine.

Trying to bridge the gulf

When we seek to bridge the gulf of not knowing, in order to know some-one more deeply, what can we draw upon to help us?

Personal experience may help a bit. But this is not always as useful as we might wish. What we have discovered from our own experience, or learned from the experience of others, can only take us so far towards getting to know somebody who is new to us.[2] Experience can help us to relate familiar to familiar, but it cannot familiarize us with what is not yet known.

---

2 Bion used to remind us that we do not know the patient of today, as we cannot (yet) know where the patient has been since the last session or where the patient is today. So, in this sense, each patient is new to us *each* day.

We are sometimes confronted by a patient whose life experience, in some significant way, appears to have been similar to our own. This might appear as an advantage. But there are dangers in this, as we can be tempted to read a patient too much in terms of our own experience.

The opposite can also happen, when a patient complains that we are not able to understand, on the grounds that we have *not* been through something similar. For instance, how can a male analyst begin to comprehend a childless woman's experience of loss through an early hysterectomy? In fact, he can never adequately comprehend this. But there may yet be something to be gained from knowing, at least, that he does not know. He therefore has to stretch his imagination, even to begin to grasp this, whereas a female analyst who has been through some similar experience may too readily imagine that she knows more than she does of what the patient is going through. One person's experience of that loss is not necessarily the same as another's. We therefore need to remember that the suffering of another person will always (in some sense) be beyond our own experience; and we need to respect this fact in order to remain open to learning more from the person concerned.

There are gains and losses in both situations. When experience provides us with the illusion of having a short cut to understanding, there may be much that is being missed. On the other hand, when we face the limitations to any generalizing from our own experience it can become more evident that there remains a significant gulf of not-knowing. The skills of empathic imagination and trial-identification will then be seen as all the more important.

The otherness of the other

It is striking just how different another person's experience can be from our own. Annie Sullivan, a teacher of the deaf and the blind, was asked to work with Helen Keller (who was deaf, blind and mute) and they eventually managed to communicate. It is, however, shockingly easy to note those three simple adjectives (deaf, blind, mute) which are used to describe Helen Keller, without fully taking in the stark fact that she could not hear, she could not see, and she could not speak.

> Annie Sullivan (portrayed as the 'Miracle Worker' in the play of that name) could only imagine what the private world of this frightened child might be. Helen Keller had lived in a world of objects that she could only touch, taste or smell. Some objects were hard, some were soft; some were cold, some were warm; some were motionless,

while others moved. And among those that moved was one that sometimes clung to her and frightened her. *That* was Helen's mother.

Before meeting Annie Sullivan, Helen had been limited to whatever sense of the world she alone could create, in the absence of any more normal means of communication. She had been limited to non-verbal communication. However, with one person (another child) she had developed a system of signals to mean 'give me' or 'you take'. That seems to have been about the extent of communication she had achieved with anyone. So she must have had the impression that hardly anyone was able to understand her at all. And, for most of the time, her frightened mother could not understand her either.

The nearly insuperable task of trying to communicate with this almost unknowable child will be clear to anyone who gives thought to it. And it had seemed to be impossible until Annie Sullivan came on the scene. But no fuller communication was possible until a bridge of understanding between Annie and Helen had been achieved.

What paved the way was when Helen recovered an extremely early memory (from the time before her hearing had finally ceased) in remembering the word 'water'. She was then able to make links between *water from the garden pump* and *this remembered word*. And, beyond that, she was also able to link this with the *pattern of letters being spelled out on her hand*.

With Annie Sullivan's help, upon this single structure was built Helen's realization that objects had names; and that these names, and the letters that were used to spell them, could become the basis for communication. Thus, having found that connection, this previously unknowable child could begin to be known; and she could also begin to relate to others.

The above example is so unusual that none of us is ever likely to meet anything like it. But it serves to exercise our imagination in the task of trying to get to know someone whose experience has been very different from our own.

However, our problem is usually not so much that of knowing that we do not know; rather it is often the *illusion* of knowing when we do not.

An extended example

To a lesser extent I too have had to get to know a patient whose early childhood, like that of Helen Keller, was absolutely different from anything I had known. I will now describe two sequences from the second year of an analysis with a patient I shall call Mr F.

For reasons of confidentiality I will not be giving much of the background history, but the most relevant detail from this patient's childhood is that he was born so short-sighted (unable to focus at a distance greater than 2 cm) that he could not see the world around him. He could not even see his mother's face. And it was not until he was aged three and a half that his parents allowed themselves to realize that he was nearly blind.

The patient was in his early twenties when he first came to see me. In the second year of his analysis there were some occasions when I could not identify, even approximately, what Mr F was trying to communicate to me. At such times he was often being elliptical in what he was saying, so that none of it seemed to come into a proper focus for me. Eventually, I realized that it was as if I were being drawn into something of his own experience of not being able to see, which I began to understand in terms of *projective identification*. Therefore, when this was happening again, I said to him:

> There are times, like today, when I have had to realize that I cannot understand what you are saying. I am not sure whether this is because I am really missing something, or whether it may be that you are somehow communicating to me something of *your* experience of not being able to see clearly.

Mr F became deeply moved. He had been experiencing me as the parents who were blind to the fact that he was almost blind, particularly when I had been trying to interpret to him in ways that were more familiar to me. Now that I was beginning to see the limits to my own way of seeing, he began to feel that I was more in touch with him and with his experience.

Comment

As well as my picking up the *projective identification* of the patient's experience of not being able to see, I think I was also picking up some *unconscious role-responsiveness* (Sandler, 1976) of the parents, who were not seeing clearly. Therefore, so long as I remained silent on this, I was probably experienced by Mr F as just like his parents, who were not acknowledging their failure to understand his disability. (Instead of recognizing his near-blindness they had been thinking that he was being clumsy, stupid or even that he might be an 'idiot' child.) But when I admitted that I had not been able to recognize what he had been trying to communicate to me, this changed. Mr F then began to experience me now as able to be in touch with him.

Shortly after this there was another occasion when Mr F was speaking in this strange way. He then said:

> My words are not other people's words, and their words are not mine. They only sound the same. (Pause.) A dog is not a dog. *Why is a cat not a dog?* (Long pause.)

Not surprisingly, I could not understand this. Mr F went on to describe how he had come to learn names for objects. For him, it had not been a process of naming objects (as for most children) but one of trying to locate objects to which he could attach the names he had already learned. He did not have any of the usual experience of a child saying: 'Mummy, what is that?' Instead his mother would say things like: 'Look, a cat', which of course he could not see. I said:

> I think you are telling me about the times when my interpretations have not matched with your experience. I am still having to learn your language, through a better understanding of your experience, and through getting to know how different this has been for you from what I might otherwise have imagined.

The patient then told me about what he described as a 'hidden breakdown' that he had when he was 16. He had come to realize he had two languages. To other people they sounded the same, but they were not the same for him. Both languages appeared to be the same, and had the same words, but the words meant completely different things for him. He had wanted to tell his parents that their language was not his, but he had been afraid they would think he was mad. His own language had 'full' words, but when he used his parents' language it seemed to him that he was using 'empty' words. He said he could never explain this to anyone, as he felt sure they would not have understood.

Mr F then elaborated that the words he had first learned, when he could not see, were the words that described his experiences of discovery. For instance, he could not know immediately whether a shape that moved was a cat or a dog. He had to find ways of working out which it was. Similarly, whenever he took an object into his hands, it was through touch and smell that he would learn to identify it. But when he was given glasses he had to name everything again – naming objects that were now visible. The names then given to objects were the same as he had used before, but the 'new' names had no sense of discovery about them. They merely attached names to objects, now they could be seen, thus by-passing the whole process of having to work out what an object was.

So when other people used names for objects they were speaking of their own experience of identifying what they could see. Previously, he had no way of communicating his quite different experience of having had to work things out for himself. But he could sense, from my response to what he was telling me, that I was now beginning to understand the difference for him, between his inner language of *discovery* and the external language of *naming*. He became deeply moved by my being able to understand this. Shortly after, Mr F had a dream.

> In this dream he had gone to see a new house with his wife and two children. At first he was concerned that the house would not be suitable. There was no bedroom for the children near enough to the parents' bedroom, so they might call out in the night and not be heard. Then he found a room he had not seen before, which was just right. It was next door to the parental room. The house now seemed to be exactly what they were looking for.

The dream continued:

> Downstairs was an amazing room. It had a huge french window looking out onto a garden and *the garden came right into the house*.

When associating to the dream Mr F spoke first of his experience in the analysis, in which he felt I had helped him to find a place for the child in himself, near enough to a parent-person who could hear his cries of distress. He was beginning to feel more secure now. He no longer felt so isolated. Mr F then spoke about the garden room, saying:

> The garden formed a bridge between the inside and the outside. Your understanding of the two languages has provided a bridge.

I added:

> Yes, a bridge between your internal world, which includes the isolated world of your early years, and the world of others.

He agreed enthusiastically. And, since then, Mr F has referred to this finding of a bridge as one of the most fundamental things achieved in his analysis.

Much of what followed from that time in the analysis focused on Mr F's experience that no one had been in touch with what he had been going through during his early years. But his finding that I had begun to be in touch with his early world also led to difficulties, as it highlighted what had been missing for him in his childhood, when it really did seem that nobody understood the nature of the world that he lived in. He was deeply relieved I could understand, but he also found it extremely painful. I believe this was because of what I have come to think of as *the pain of contrast*.

Comment

I have quite often noticed that patients can feel profoundly distressed in the midst of good experience. Some analysts interpret this too readily in terms of *envy*, or more specifically as *negative therapeutic reaction*, which in turn is usually understood as a manifestation of envy. And yet it seems to me that, at times, there may be a quite different explanation of this apparently negative response. When a patient experiences something good with the analyst it can *by contrast* bring home how much this kind of good experience may have been missing in the patient's childhood. It can be extremely painful to discover, and to experience, what has previously been missing.

An interesting outcome of this analysis was found to be in a different emphasis on the nature of interpretation, at least in this part of my work with Mr F that I have described here. For instance, when I tried to interpret something he did not see for himself, Mr F often experienced this as if I were trying to shift him away from his own unfocused world into a world where value is given to seeing things more clearly. But this was confusingly close to his experience of his parents, who had seemed to be so consistently denying the reality of his blurred world while they tried to get him to see things as they saw them. The irony here had been that his parents, in trying to introduce him to their external world, were at the same time denying his experience of the world as he knew it.

For quite some time, therefore, it was necessary for me to be prepared to relax my preference for seeing things clearly, so that I could be drawn by my patient into his blurred world, and to the quite different reality he experienced there.

It was in that unfocused world he had learned the names for objects, which he could only dimly discern. And in that blurred world, a shape that moved in a certain way could at first be either a cat or a dog. Only gradually could he distinguish one from the other. And when he could do that, it had been an important achievement for him. Therefore, *his* words 'cat' and 'dog' had been the names he had given to the whole process of discovery, and these were what he had come to think of as 'full words'. But the names 'cat' and 'dog', in the sighted world, came to mean something very different for him. Other people used these words to name what they could see, whereas when he used them in that way these were *for him* just 'empty words'. There was no sense of discovery about them.

The gains for this patient, in his analysis, were not just those in which I had been able to interpret what he could not understand on his own. What he seems to have valued far more was the extent to which I had been able to learn the language of his pre-sighted world, and his discovery with me that he could communicate what he seems never to have been able to communicate to anyone before.

The unknown beyond the known

I am reminded of what Bollas wrote in his first book *The Shadow of the Object*:

> There is in each of us a fundamental split between *what we think we know and what we know but may never be able to think*. In the course of the transference and countertransference the psychoanalyst may be able to facilitate the transfer of the unthought known into thought, and the patient will come to put into thought something about his being which he has not been able to think up until then.
>
> (Bollas, 1987: 282)

In that passage he is writing mainly of the unknown in the patient. In this chapter I have been more concerned with *that which remains unknown to the analyst*, and what can happen when analysts fail to recognize that which lies beyond their own experience or understanding.

Of course, analysts are trained not to put onto patients what does not belong to them. In particular they are trained not to attribute to patients what may belong to themselves, or to use patients as transferential objects. But it is not so much from the analyst's personal experience, or feelings, that some patients can be at risk so much as *from what may be transferred or projected onto them from other clinical experience – or from theory*. I think of this mistaken use of theory, or of one's own experience, as another kind of transference (from the analyst): some understanding from elsewhere is being put onto a patient that does not necessarily apply. The problem here is that practice wisdom naturally accrues from clinical experience, and yet this can result in sometimes not recognizing when this understanding from elsewhere could be misapplied.

Though careful not to fall into the more typical forms of transference or projection, analysts can nevertheless develop a false sense of confidence in their theoretical framework and in the broad applicability of their clinical experience. Of course, in any analysis, there is an essential place for theory and for clinical experience, but for some analysts (and I count myself among them) that remains secondary to the task of trying to get to understand the individual. I therefore hope not to allow myself to be pushed into seeing a patient in any particular way just because theory (or someone else) suggests that I should. Each patient is essentially unique. The individual will therefore still remain something of a mystery, however well we may eventually come to know him/her. Therefore, even though theory has a vital place in serving the work of analysis I continue to hope we will not be governed by it too often.

The value of not-knowing

Winnicott, in particular, kept reminding us of the importance of sustaining a level of not-knowing in relation to patients we are still trying to get to know, which means every patient throughout every analysis.[3] And, in his own way, so did Bion.

> Instead of trying to bring a brilliant, intelligent, knowledgeable light to bear on obscure problems, I suggest we bring to bear a diminution of the 'light' – a penetrating beam of darkness; a reciprocal of the searchlight . . . The darkness would be so absolute that it would achieve a luminous, absolute vacuum. So that, if any object existed, however faint, it would show up very clearly. Thus, a very faint light would become visible in maximum conditions of darkness.
>
> (Bion 1974: 37)

Some patients come into analysis with shattering experiences locked in their minds, or with inconceivable chaos and confusion spilling into consciousness. If analysts are truly to engage with these experiences, rather than defending themselves with familiar theory, they need to look

---

3 I understand that cognitive psychologists are working with a similar concept these days, namely that a clinician should be willing to challenge his or her own assumptions, to test and re-test the hypotheses he or she has formed, and adjust the case conceptualization accordingly – on almost a continuous basis. For example, see Beck (1995) and Persons (1989).

for that faint light of meaning in the midst of all that may seem like non-sense. And some things presented by the patient may threaten to be upsetting also for the analyst, disturbing the analyst's view of himself/herself or his preconceptions about theory or technique.

For instance, it may be the primitive registration of early trauma that requires fresh understanding, even though it could defy established theories of memory. Maybe we have to take more seriously a notion of body memory to make sense of this.[4] Or, we may be faced by details of trauma that we would much prefer to regard as unbelievable, such as the extremes of sexual abuse that have been described as 'satanic'. It is much more comfortable for the analyst to cling to theories of unconscious phantasy, or to diagnose psychosis in the patient, than to dare to believe that *occasionally* there may be some truth in these terrible accounts of abuse.[5] And, at the opposite extreme, it may be ineffable experience (religious and/or spiritual) that should prompt us to wonder whether psychoanalytic theory can really explain *all* of this away. In situations such as these, we may encounter areas of experience that go beyond anything that we have any direct knowledge of, or adequate theory to encompass.

Equally, we may find ourselves used by a patient in ways that go beyond what we regard as proper to an analysis, or in ways that profoundly test our usual technique. For instance, I was persuaded by one patient (for quite long periods) not to interpret at all. Instead, I listened (mostly in silence) for session after session, hardly being allowed to speak, and then being allowed only to register that I had recognized some essence of what I was being told. It felt very strange and as if I was being rendered entirely impotent. And some might say that I had colluded with the controlling demands of my patient. But the analysis continued and later began to prove to have been more fruitful than when I had still imagined that I should be

---

4   At the time of first writing this chapter I was not familiar with the comparatively new notion of *implicit memory*. Of this Regina writes: 'If declarative/explicit memory is the memory for the aspects of experience of which we are conscious, then by contrast non-declarative, also called implicit, memory is the memory for the aspects of experience that are non-consciously processed ... What this means is that certain information can be stored in memory without our having been consciously aware of its occurrence; it can non-consciously influence current functioning but does not feel like conscious remembering. Implicit memory includes the memory for shape and form (primed memory), emotion (emotional memory) and skills, habits and routines (procedural memory), each of which is processed in a different brain system' (1997: 1228).

5   See also 'On the wish not to know' (Casement, 1994).

the one to provide understanding. And it is not insignificant that this patient's mother was profoundly deaf.

Conclusion

I have only been able to approach the title of this chapter indirectly. Of course we cannot know 'the unknown' before we meet it. My point is that we may never meet it in analysis if we approach the analytic task *only* in terms of what we already know. The best we can do, therefore, is to recognize the problems that stem from knowledge, whether that is based upon our experience of life, our clinical experience, or our training. Sometimes it is beyond all of this that the unknown of a patient lies, especially when it does not fit with what we have previously known. But when that unknown is found to have the 'light' that Bion speaks of, *a light that does not come from the analyst but from the patient*, we have something important to learn from it.

Finally, if we really engage with something previously unknown to us *we are changed by it*. This is because we are challenged by it. We are challenged in how we view ourselves, in how we view the patient, in how we view our theory and our technique. If we resist that challenge we may miss the significance of whatever threatens our present thinking. And what might we be doing to a patient, who needs us to risk being extended in how we think and how we work, if we cannot meet them openly in areas of experience for which we do not yet have any adequate map?

However, if we are careful to follow the patient, and do not attempt to lead, we can afford to venture beyond the familiar. We can even risk getting out of our depth, and sometimes getting lost, until we later discover where we have got to and where we have been. And, if we are willing to learn from patients such as Mr F, we have much to learn in the realm that lies beyond what we already know. We may then become better able to move beyond our merely giving names to what we can more readily see, in that process which we otherwise call interpretation.

Epilogue
Getting where?

Are we getting near to where patients most need us to get?

- Who benefits most from psychoanalysis? Is it the patient or might it sometimes be the analyst?
- Are we in danger of using patients to give credence to our theories rather than remaining sufficiently open to the individuality of each patient, with theory remaining our servant rather than this becoming our master?
- When we are considering a patient's response to our interpretations, how readily do we look beyond the content of what we have been saying? Might a patient be responding less to *what* we are saying and more to *how* we are saying it?
- To what extent is psychic change due to interpretation, bringing the unconscious to conscious awareness, and to what extent might it be due to the patient's experience of the analytic relationship?
- What part does the analytic relationship itself play in bringing about change? In so far as the relationship is found to benefit the patient, to what extent is this a central factor in the analytic process and to what extent is it just a by-product of that process?
- When a patient opposes the analyst, is this always to be regarded as resistance or an attack on the analysis; or might it sometimes be an attempt to be understood better?
- When a patient is late, is this always to be seen as resistance or might it sometimes be that the patient is coming in his/her own time rather than at a time set by the analyst? If so, is that necessarily a bad thing or might there, at times, be something positive in it?
- Does 'being taken for granted' by a patient always have to be something contemptuous? Might it not sometimes be an act of trust?
- If a patient refuses to use the couch, or gets off the couch, is this

necessarily to be regarded as resistance or might the patient be needing to work differently, at least for a time?

- When we interpret some acting out, are we trying to stop it through interpretation or are we trying to understand it?
- When we hear of a colleague getting caught into some enactment, do we usually assume that this is indicating a countertransference problem in the other or can we also allow for an unconscious interplay between the patient and analyst, which might be better understood as part of the analytic process?
- When we see others as apparently mistaken in how they work, could it be that they are sometimes in touch with aspects of this difficult work that we ourselves may not yet be seeing?
- When there are opposing ways of seeing clinical material, does one way have to be seen as right and any other as wrong? Could there be valuable elements in each?
- If there is a divide between different kinds of analysis, is one kind being more true to psychoanalysis than the other? If so, which one is being more true? And can we still learn from each other across this divide? Or should there be a parting of the ways, so that each can develop more freely into the clinical practice that each has the potential to become?
- Is psychoanalysis still to be regarded as a science? If so, what kind of a science? Is it not possible that quite serious misconceptions have arisen as a result of analysts being too ready to apply analytic notions universally when it may be necessary to remain more tuned into the individual, and being more cautious?
- Are analysts sufficiently careful in their use of authority, whether in the consulting room or outside it, in claiming to understand their patients, or life, more deeply than others?
- Are analysts ready to accept those times when they could be mistaken? Or do they continue to assume that error belongs mostly to others rather than to themselves?
- When things go well in an analysis do we give sufficient credit to the patient for their part in this, or do we take most of the credit for ourselves? And when things go badly do we accept responsibility for our own part in this or do we mostly blame the patient for it?

These are just some of the questions that may help us to avoid complacency about our theories and ways of working. There are of course many others. But the overriding questions for me have been:

- Are we finding ways that truly free the mind and creativity of those who come to us for analysis or therapy?
- Do we adequately guard against the danger of turning others into some version of our own selves, so that they then come to see themselves as we have been seeing them?

I believe that such questions as these are most fruitful if they are kept open, still challenging us. And we lose something important if we seek to protect ourselves by too readily assuming that we can answer them.

Appendix

Some pressures on the analyst for physical contact during the reliving of an early trauma[1]

Is physical contact with the patient, even of a token kind, always to be precluded without question under the classical rule of abstinence? Or are there some occasions when this might be appropriate, even necessary, as Margaret Little has suggested in relation to episodes of delusional transference (1957, 1958) or as Balint and Winnicott have illustrated in relation to periods of deep regression (e.g. Balint, 1952, 1968; Winnicott, 1954a, 1963a)?

I shall present a clinical sequence during which the possibility of physical contact was approached as an open issue. There seemed to be a case for allowing a patient the possibility of holding my hand. The decision to reconsider this was arrived at from listening to the patient and from following closely the available cues from the countertransference. The clinical material clearly illustrates some of the issues involved in this decision.

The patient, whom I shall call Mrs B, is in her thirties. She had been in analysis about two and a half years. A son had been born during the second year of the analysis.

When she was 11 months old Mrs B had been severely scalded, having pulled boiling water onto herself while her mother was out of the room. She could have died from the burns. When she was 17 months old she had to be operated on to release growing skin from the dead scar tissue. The operation was done under a local anaesthetic. During this the mother had fainted. (It is relevant to the childhood history that the father was largely absent during the first five years.)

Soon after the summer holiday Mrs B presented the following dream. *She had been trying to feed a despairing child. The child was standing*

1 Reprinted from *International Review of Psycho-Analysis* 9: 279–286.

and was about 10 months old. It wasn't clear whether the child was a boy or a girl. Mrs B wondered about the age of the child. Her son was soon to be 10 months old. He was now able to stand. She too would have been standing at 10 months. (That would have been before the accident.) Why was the child in her dream so despairing, she asked. Her son is a lively child and she assumed that she too had been a normal happy child until the accident. This prompted me to recall how Mrs B had clung to an idealized view of her pre-accident childhood. I thought she was now daring to question this. I therefore commented that maybe she was beginning to wonder about the time before the accident. Perhaps not everything had been quite so happy as she had always needed to assume. She immediately held up her hand to signal me to stop.

During the following silence I wondered why there was this present anxiety. Was it the patient's need still not to look at anything from before the accident unless it was seen as perfect? Was the accident itself being used as a screen memory? I thought this probable. After a while I said that she seemed to be afraid of finding any element of bad experience during the time before the accident, as if she still felt that the good that had been there before must be kept entirely separate from the bad that had followed. She listened in silence, making no perceptible response during the rest of the session.

The next day Mrs B came to her session with a look of terror on her face. For this session, and the five sessions following, she could not lie on the couch. She explained that when I had gone on talking, after she had signalled me to stop, the couch had 'become' the operating table with me as the surgeon, who had gone on operating regardless, after her mother had fainted. She now couldn't lie down 'because the experience will go on'. Nothing could stop it then, she felt sure. In one of these sitting-up sessions Mrs B showed me a photograph of her holiday house, built into the side of a mountain with high retaining walls. She stressed how essential these walls are to hold the house from falling. She was afraid of falling for ever.[2] She felt this had happened to her after her mother had fainted.

(Here I should mention that Mrs B had previously recalled thinking that her mother had died, when she had fallen out of her sight during the operation, and how she had felt that she was left alone with no one to

---

2 'Falling for ever' is referred to by Winnicott as one of the 'unthinkable anxieties' along with 'going to pieces', 'having no relationship to the body' and 'having no orientation' (1962: 58).

protect her from the surgeon who seemed to be about to kill her with his knife.) Now, in this session, Mrs B told me a detail of that experience which she had never mentioned before. At the start of the operation her mother had been holding her hands in hers, and Mrs B remembered her terror upon finding her mother's hands slipping out of hers as she fainted and disappeared. She now thought she had been trying to re-find her mother's hands ever since, and she began to stress the importance of physical contact for her. She said she couldn't lie down on the couch again unless she knew she could, if necessary, hold my hand in order to get through the reliving of the operation experience. Would I allow this or would I refuse? If I refused she wasn't sure that she could continue with her analysis.

My initial response was to acknowledge to her that she needed me to be 'in touch' with the intensity of her anxiety. However, she insisted that she had to know whether or not I would actually allow her to hold my hand. I felt under increased pressure due to this being near the end of a Friday session, and I was beginning to fear that the patient might indeed leave the analysis. My next comment was defensively equivocal. I said that some analysts would not contemplate allowing this, but I realized that she might need to have the possibility of holding my hand if it seemed to be the only way for her to get through this experience. She showed some relief upon my saying this.[3]

Over the weekend I reviewed the implications of this possibility of the patient holding my hand. While reflecting upon my countertransference around this issue I came to recognize the following key points: (1) I was in effect offering to be the 'better mother' who would remain holding her hand, in contrast to the actual mother who had not been able to bear what was happening. (2) My offer had been partly motivated by my fear of losing this patient, which was especially threatening to me just then as I was about to present a paper on this patient to our Society. (3) If I were to hold this patient's hand it would almost certainly not, as she assumed, help her to get through a re-experiencing of the original trauma. (A central factor of this had been the absence of her mother's hands.) It would instead amount to a by-passing of this aspect of the trauma, and could reinforce the patient's perception of this as something too terrible ever fully to be remembered or to be experienced. I therefore decided that I must review with the patient the implications of this offer as soon as I had an opportunity to do so.

3 At the time I was thinking that this offer of the possibility of holding my hand might, in Eissler's (1953) terms, be a permissible 'parameter'.

On the Sunday I received a hand-delivered letter in which the patient said she had had another dream of the despairing child, but this time there were signs of hope. *The child was crawling towards a motionless figure with the excited expectation of reaching this figure.*

On the Monday, although she was somewhat reassured by her dream, Mrs B remained sitting on the couch. She saw the central figure as me representing her missing mother. She also stressed that she hadn't wanted me to have to wait to know about the dream. I interpreted her fear that I might not have been able to wait to be reassured, and she agreed. She had been afraid that I might have collapsed over the weekend, under the weight of the Friday session, if I had been left until Monday without knowing that she was beginning to feel more hopeful.

As this session continued, what emerged was a clear impression that Mrs B was seeing the possibility of holding my hand as a 'short-cut' to feeling safer. She wanted me to be the motionless figure, controlled by her and not allowed to move, towards whom she could crawl with the excited expectation that she would eventually be allowed to touch me. Mrs B then reported an image, which was a continuation in the session of the written dream. She saw the dream-child reaching the central figure, but as she touched this it had crumbled and collapsed. With this cue as my lead I told her that I had thought very carefully about this, and I had come to the conclusion that this tentative offer of my hand might have appeared to provide a way of getting through the experience she was so terrified of, but I now realized that it would instead become a side-stepping of that experience as it had been rather than a living through it. I knew that if I seemed to be inviting an avoidance of this central aspect of the original experience I would be failing her as her analyst. I therefore did not think that I should leave the possibility of holding my hand still open to her. Mrs B looked stunned. She asked me if I realized what I had just done. I had taken my hand away from her just as her mother had, and she immediately assumed that this must be because I too couldn't bear to remain in touch with what she was going through. Nothing I said could alter her assumption that I was afraid to let her touch me.

The following day the patient's response to what I had said was devastating. Still sitting on the couch she told me that her left arm (the one nearest to me) was 'steaming'. I had burned her. She couldn't accept any interpretation from me. Only a real physical response from me could do anything about it. She wanted to stop her analysis to get away from what was happening to her in her sessions. She could never trust me again. I tried to interpret that her trust in her mother, which had in a fragile way been restored after the accident, seemed to have been finally broken after her mother had fainted. It was this ultimate breach of her trust in her mother that had got in the way of her subsequent relationship to her. I felt it was this that she was now in the process of re-enacting with me in order to find that this unresolved breach of trust could be repaired. She listened to this, and was nodding understanding, but she repeated that it was impossible to repair.

The following day Mrs B raged at me still for what she saw as my withdrawing from her. The possibility of holding my hand had been the same to her as actual holding. She felt sure she would not have abused the offer. It had been vitally important to her that I had been prepared to allow this, but my change of mind had become to her a real dropping away of the hand she needed to hold on to. To her I was now her mother who had become afraid. Her arm seemed to be on fire. To her I was afraid of being burned too.

Mrs B told me that the previous day, immediately after her session with me, she had become 'fully suicidal'. She had only got out of this by asking a friend if she could go round to see her, at any time, if she felt that she couldn't carry on. She hadn't ultimately needed to see her friend. It had been her friend's availability which had prevented her from killing herself. She then rebuked me with the fact that her friend could get it right. Why couldn't I? I told her that she did not need from me what she could get from others. She needed something different from me. She needed me not to buy off her anger by offering to be the 'better mother'. It was important that I should not be afraid of her anger, or of her despair, in order that I stay with her throughout the relived experience of no longer having her mother's hands to hold on to. She needed me to remain analyst rather than have me as a 'pretend' mother. It was also crucial that I do nothing that could suggest that I needed to protect myself from what she was experiencing or was feeling towards me. She listened and became calmer. Then, momentarily before leaving the session, she lay down on the couch. She thus resumed the lying position.

I shall now summarize the next two weeks. Mrs B dreamed of being lost and unsafe amongst a strange people with whom she could not find a common language. I interpreted her anxiety as to whether I could find a common language with her. In one session she had a visual image of a child crying stone tears, which I interpreted as the tears of a petrified child (herself). She dreamed of *a baby being dropped and left to die*. She dreamed of *being very small and being denied the only food she wanted. It was there but a tall person would not let her have it*. In another dream *she was in terror anticipating some kind of explosion*. Throughout this she persisted in her conviction that she could never trust me again, and she experienced me as afraid of her. Alongside this she told me that her husband had become very supporting of her continuing her analysis, even though he was getting a lot of 'kick-back' from it. This was quite new. I interpreted that at some level she was becoming more aware of me as able to take the kick-back from her, in her analysis.

Shortly after this Mrs B reported the following two dreams in the same session. In the first *she was taking a child every day to meet her mother to get some order into the chaos*, which I interpreted as her bringing her child-self to me in order to work through the chaos of her feelings towards me as the mother she still couldn't trust. She agreed with this but added that she didn't bring the child to me by the hand. She had to drag her child-self by the hair. In the second dream *she was falling through the air, convinced that she was going to die despite the fact that she was held by a parachute with a helicopter watching over her*. She could see the contradictions (sure of dying whilst actually being safe) but this did not stop her feeling terrified in the dream, and still terrified of me in the session. She stressed that she didn't know if I realized that she was still feeling sure that she was dying inside.

On the following Monday Mrs B told me that she had dreamed that *she had come for her last session as she couldn't go on. She had begun falling for ever, the couch and the room falling with her. There was no bottom and no end to it.*

The next day the patient felt that she was going insane. She had dreamed *there was a sheet of glass between herself and me so that she couldn't touch me or see me clearly. It was like a car windscreen with no wipers in a storm.* I interpreted her inability to feel that I could get in touch with what she was feeling, because of the barrier between her and me created by the storm of her feelings inside her. This prevented her seeing me clearly, just as it had with her mother. She agreed and collapsed into uncontrolled crying, twisting on the couch, tortured with pain. At the end of this session she became panicked that I wouldn't be able to tolerate having experienced this degree of her distress.

On the Friday she spoke of a new worker in her office. She had asked him how long he had been trained. She then realized that she was asking him for his credentials. I interpreted her anxiety about my credentials and whether I had the necessary experience to be able to see her through. I added that maybe she used the word 'credentials' because of the allusion to 'believe'. She replied 'Of course, credo.' She said that she wanted to believe that I could see her through, and to trust me, but she still couldn't.

The next week Mrs B continued to say that she didn't think she could go on. She had had many terrible dreams over the weekend. The following day she again sat up for the session. For much of this session she seemed to be quite deluded. Awareness of reality was fleeting and tenuous. For the greater part of the session she was a child. She began by saying she didn't just talk to her baby, she picks him up and holds him. Then, looking straight at me she said 'I am a baby and you are the person I need to be my mother. I need you to realize this, because unless you are prepared to hold me I cannot go on. You have got to understand this.' She was putting me under immense pressure. Finally she stared accusingly at me and said 'You *are* my mother and you are *not* holding me.'

Throughout this I was aware of the delusional quality of her perception of me.[4] In this session there was little 'as if' sense left in her experience of me, and at times there seemed to be none. It was meaningless to her when I attempted to interpret this as transference, as a reliving of her childhood experience. Not only was I the mother who was not holding her, in her terror of me I had also become the surgeon with a knife in his hand who seemed to be about to kill her. At this point there seemed to be no remaining contact with me as analyst.

I reflected upon my dilemma. If I did *not* give in to her demands I might lose the patient, or she might really go psychotic and need to be hospitalized. If I *did* give in to her I would be colluding with her delusional perception of me, and the avoided elements of the trauma could become encapsulated as too terrible ever to confront. I felt placed in an impossible position. However, once I came to recognize the projective identification process operating here I began to surface from this feeling of complete helplessness. This enabled me eventually to interpret from my counter-transference feelings. Very slowly, and with pauses to check that the patient was following me, I said to her 'You are making me experience in myself the sense of despair, and the impossibility of going on, that you are feeling. I am aware of being in what feels to me like a total paradox. In one sense I am feeling that it is impossible to reach you just now, and yet in another sense I feel that my telling you this may be the only way I can reach you.' She followed what I was saying very carefully, and slightly nodded her head. I continued, 'Similarly I feel as if it could be impossible to go on, and yet I feel that the only way I can help you through this is by my being prepared to tolerate what you are making me feel, and going on.' After a long silence Mrs B began to speak to me again as analyst. She said 'For the first time I can believe you, that you are in touch with what I have been feeling, and what is so amazing is that you can bear

---

4 I now understand this in terms of the psychic immediacy of the transference experience.

it.' I was then able to interpret to her that her desperate wish for me to let her touch me had been her way of letting me know that she needed me to be really in touch with what she was going through. This time she could agree. She remained in silence for the last 10 minutes of this session, and I sensed that it was important that I should do nothing to interrupt this in any way.

The following day Mrs B told me what had been happening during that silence. She had been able to smell her mother's presence, and she had felt her mother's hands again holding hers. She felt that it was her mother from before the fainting that she had got in touch with, as she had never felt held like that since then. I commented that she had been able to find the internal mother that she had lost touch with, as distinct from the 'pretend' mother she had been wanting me to become. We could now see that if I had agreed to hold her physically it would have been a way of shutting off what she was experiencing, not only for her but also for me, as if I really couldn't bear to remain with her through this. She immediately recognized the implications of what I was saying and replied, 'Yes. You would have become a collapsed analyst. I could not realize it at the time but I can now see that you would then have become the same as my mother who fainted. I am so glad you didn't let that happen.'

To conclude I will summarize part of the last session in this week. Mrs B had woken feeling happy and had later found herself singing extracts from the opera *Der Freischütz*, the plot of which (she explained) includes the triumph of light over darkness. She had also dreamed that *she was in a car which had got out of control having taken on a life of its own. The car crashed into a barrier which had prevented her from running into the oncoming traffic. The barrier had saved her because it had remained firm. If it had collapsed she would have been killed.* She showed great relief that I had withstood her angry demands. My remaining firm had been able to stop the process which had taken on a life of its own, during which she had felt completely out of control. The same dream ended with *the patient reaching out to safety through the car windscreen which had opened to her like two glass doors.*

Discussion

This case illustrates the interplay between the various dynamics operating. My initial offer of possible physical contact was, paradoxically, tantamount to the countertransference withdrawal which the patient later attributed to me in my decision not to leave this offer of that easier option open to her. In terms of Bion's (1962) concept of 'a projective-identification-rejecting-object' the countertransference here became *the container's fear of the contained*. A further complicating pressure came from the fact that I was shortly to present a paper on this patient to our Society, and I was genuinely afraid of being exposed there as having failed had my patient left the analysis, or had she needed to be hospitalized, just prior to my presenting that paper concerning her. By offering the possibility of the patient holding my hand I was in effect seeking to lessen these risks to myself, and this is an example of Racker's (1968) concept of *indirect countertransference*, in that my response to the patient here was being influenced by some degree of persecutory superego being projected by me on to my professional colleagues.

The resulting sequence can be understood in the interactional terms of Sandler's (1976) concept of *role-responsiveness* or in terms of Winnicott's description of the patient's need to be able to experience in the present, in relation to a real situation between patient and analyst, the extremes of feeling which belonged to an early traumatic experience but which had been 'frozen' because of being too intense for the primitive ego to encompass *at that time* (Winnicott, 1954b, 1963b; see also Winnicott, 1974). There had come to be a real issue between this patient and me, in the withdrawal of my earlier offer of the possibility of holding my hand. In using this to represent the central element of the original trauma the patient entered into an intensely real experience of the past as she had perceived it. In so doing she was able, as it were, to 'join up with' her own feelings, now unfrozen and available to her. The repressed past became, in the present, a conscious psychic reality from which (this time) she did not have defensively to be psychically absent. During this I had to continue to be the surviving analyst, and not become a collapsed analyst, in order that she could defuse the earlier phantasy that it had been the intensity of her need for her mother that had caused her mother to faint.

The eventual interpretive resolution within this session grew out of my awareness of the *projective identification process* then operating. I am understanding this here as the product of interactional pressures upon the analyst, from the patient, which are unconsciously aiming to evoke in him the unbearable feeling state which the patient could not on her own yet contain within herself (cf. Ogden, 1979). It is a matter for speculation whether I would have been so fully subjected to the necessary impact of this patient's experience had I not first approached the question of possible physical contact as an open issue. Had I gone by the book, following the classical rule of no physical contact under any circumstance, I would certainly have been taking the safer course for me but I would probably then have been accurately perceived by the patient as actually afraid even to consider such contact. I am not sure that the reliving of this early trauma would have been as real as it was to the patient, or in the end so therapeutically effective, if I had been preserving myself throughout at that safer distance of classical 'correctness'. Instead I acted upon my intuition of the moment, and it is uncanny how precisely and unwittingly this led me to re-enact with the patient this detail of the original trauma, which she needed to be able to experience within the analytic relationship and to be genuinely angry about. It is this unconscious responsiveness to communicative cues from the patient to which Sandler refers in his (1976) paper 'Countertransference and role-responsiveness'. Winnicott also speaks of this when he says: 'In the end the patient uses the analyst's failures, often quite small ones, perhaps manoeuvred by the patient . . . and we have to put up with being in a limited context misunderstood. The operative factor is that the patient now hates the analyst for the failure that originally came as an environmental factor, outside the infant's area of omnipotent control, but that is now staged in the transference. So in the end we succeed by failing – failing the patient's way. This is a long distance from the simple theory of cure by corrective experience' (1963b: 258).

With regard to the recovered analytic holding I wish to add one further point. Because this was arrived at experientially with the patient, rather than by rule of thumb, it became more than just a proof of [a] rightness of the classical position concerning no physical contact. 'En route' this had instead acquired a specificity to this patient which, in my opinion, allowed a fuller reliving of this early trauma than might otherwise have been possible.

I shall conclude with a quotation from Bion's (1962) paper 'A theory of thinking'. He says 'If the infant *feels* [my italics] it is dying it can arouse fears that it is dying in the mother. A well-balanced mother can accept these and respond therapeutically: that is to say in a manner that makes the infant feel it is receiving its frightened personality back again but in a form that it can tolerate—the fears are manageable by the infant personality. If the mother cannot tolerate these projections the infant is reduced to continued projective identification carried out with increasing force and frequence' (pp. 114–115). Bion continues 'Normal development follows if the relationship between infant and breast permits the infant to project a feeling, say, that it is dying into the mother and to reintroject it after its sojourn in the breast has made it tolerable to the infant psyche. If the projection is not accepted by the mother the infant feels that its feeling that it is dying is stripped of such meaning as it has. It therefore reintrojects, not a fear of dying made tolerable, but a nameless dread' (p. 116).

I know that Bion is here describing an infant's relationship to the breast. Nevertheless I believe that a similar process, at a later developmental stage, is illustrated in the clinical sequence I have described. I consider that it was my readiness to preserve the restored psychoanalytical holding, in the face of considerable pressures upon me to relinquish it, which eventually enabled my patient to receive her own frightened personality back again in a form that she could tolerate. Had I resorted to the physical holding that she demanded the central trauma would have remained frozen, and could have been regarded as perhaps for ever unmanageable. The patient would then have reintrojected, not a fear of dying made tolerable, but instead a nameless dread.

Bibliography

Alexander, F., French, T.M. *et al.* (1946) The principle of corrective emotional experience, in *Psychoanalytic Therapy, Principles and Application.* New York: Ronald Press.

Aron, L. (1992) Interpretation as expression of the analyst's subjectivity. *Psychoanalytic Dialogues* 2: 475–507.

—— (1996) *A Meeting of Minds.* New York: Analytic Press.

Balint, M. (1952a) New beginning and the paranoid and depressive syndromes, in *Primary Love and Psycho-analytic Technique.* London: Tavistock Publications, 1965, pp. 230–249.

—— (1952b) *Primary Love and Psycho-analytic Technique.* London: Tavistock Publications, 1965.

—— (1968) *The Basic Fault.* London: Tavistock Publications.

Beck, J. (1995) *Cognitive Therapy: Basics and Beyond.* New York: Guilford Press.

Bion, W.R. (1962) A theory of thinking, in *Second Thoughts* (1967), New York: Jason Aronson, pp. 110–119.

—— (1967) *Second Thoughts.* New York: Jason Aronson.

—— (1974) *Brazilian Lectures 1.* Rio de Janeiro: Imago Editora.

Boesky, D. (1998) Clinical evidence and multiple models: new responsibilities. *Journal of the American Psychoanalytic Association* 46: 1013–1020.

Bollas, C. (1987) *The Shadow of the Object: Psychoanalysis of the Unthought Known.* London: Free Association Books.

Breckenridge, K. (2000) Physical touch in psychoanalysis: a closet phenomenon? *Psychoanalytic Inquiry* 20(1): 2–20.

Breuer, J. and Freud, S. (1895) Studies on hysteria. *Standard Edition* 2.

Britton, R. (1998) *Belief and Imagination: Explorations in Psychoanalysis.* London: Routledge.

Casement, P.J. (1982) Some pressures on the analyst for physical contact during the reliving of an early psychic trauma. *International Review of Psycho-Analysis* 9: 279–286.

—— (1985) *On Learning from the Patient.* London: Tavistock Publications.

—— (1990) *Further Learning from the Patient.* London: Routledge.

—— (1991) *Learning from the Patient*. New York: Guilford Press. (A combined volume that contains both *On Learning from the Patient* and *Further Learning from the Patient*.)

—— (1994) On the wish not to know, in V. Sinason (ed.), *Treating Survivors of Satanist Abuse*, London: Routledge, pp. 22–25.

—— (1998) Objective fact and psychological truth: some thoughts on 'recovered memory,' in V. Sinason (ed.), *Memory in Dispute*. London: Karnac, pp. 179–184.

—— (2000) The issue of touch: a retrospective overview. *Psychoanalytic Inquiry* 20(1): 160–184.

Chused, J.F. (1991) The evocative power of enactments. *Journal of the American Psychoanalytic Association* 39: 615–639.

—— (1997) Discussion of 'Observing-participation, mutual enactment, and the new classical models' by Irwin Hirsch, Ph.D. *Contemporary Psychoanalysis* 33: 263–77.

Chused, J.F. and Raphling, D. (1992) The analyst's mistakes. *Journal of the American Psychoanalytic Association* 40: 89–116.

Eissler, K.R. (1953) The effect of the structure of the ego on psychoanalytic technique. *Journal of the American Psychoanalytic Association* 1: 104–143.

Fiscalini, F. (1994) The uniquely interpersonal and the interpersonally unique – on interpersonal psychoanalysis. *Contemporary Psychoanalysis* 30: 114–134.

Fosshage, J.L. (2000) The meanings of touch in psychoanalysis: a time for reassessment. *Psychoanalytic Inquiry* 20(1): 21–43.

Fox, R.P. (1984) The principle of abstinence reconsidered. *International Review of Psycho-Analysis* 11: 227–236.

Freud, S. (1913) On beginning the treatment (further recommendations on the technique of psycho-analysis I). *Standard Edition* 12.

—— (1920) Beyond the pleasure principle. *Standard Edition*. 18.

Giovacchini, P.L. (ed.) (1975) *Tactics and Techniques in Psychoanalytic Therapy, Vol. 11*. New York: Jason Aronson.

Greenberg, J.R. (1986) On the analyst's neutrality. *Contemporary Psychoanalysis* 22: 87–106.

Heimann, P. (1950) On counter-transference. *International Journal of Psycho-Analysis* 31: 81–84.

Hoffer, A. (1991) The Freud-Ferenczi controversy – a living legacy. *International Review of Psycho-Analysis* 18: 465–472.

Katz, G.A. (1998) Where the action is: the enacted dimension of analytic process. *Journal of the American Psychoanalytic Association* 46: 1129–1167.

Kernberg, O. (1996) Thirty methods to destroy the creativity of psychoanalytic candidates. *International Journal of Psycho-Analysis* 77: 1031–1040.

Kirsner, D. (2000) *Unfree Associations: Inside Psychoanalytic Institutes*. London: Process Press.

Klein, M. (1946) Notes on some schizoid mechanisms, in J. Riviere (ed.), *Developments in Psycho-Analysis*. London: Hogarth Press, 1952.

Kohon, G. (ed.) (1986) *The British School of Psychoanalysis: The Independent Tradition*. London: Free Association Books.

Ladan, A. (1992) On the secret fantasy of being an exception. *International Journal of Psycho-Analysis* 73: 29–38.

Langs, R.J. (1978) *The Listening Process*. New York: Jason Aronson.

Levenson, E.A. (1992) Mistakes, errors, and oversights. *Contemporary Psychoanalysis* 28: 555–571.

Lewis, E. and Casement, P.J. (1986) The inhibition of mourning in pregnancy. *Psychoanalytic Psychotherapy* 2(1): 45–52.

Little, M. (1957) 'R' – The analyst's total response to his patient's needs. *International Journal of Psycho-Analysis* 38: 240–254.

—— (1958) On delusional transference. *International Journal of Psycho-Analysis* 39: 134–138.

Marrone, M. (1998) *Attachment and Interaction*. London and Philadelphia: Jessica Kingsley.

Meares, R.A. and Hobson, R.F. (1977) The persecutory therapist. *British Journal of Medical Psychology* 50: 349–359.

Meissner, W.W. (1996) *The Therapeutic Alliance*. New Haven, Conn.: Yale University Press.

—— (1998) Neutrality, abstinence, and the therapeutic alliance. *Journal of the American Psychoanalytic Association* 46: 1089–1128.

Mitchell, S. (1997) *Influence and Autonomy in Psychoanalysis*. Hillsdale, N.J.: Analytic Press.

Ogden, T. (1979) On projective identification. *International Journal of Psycho-Analysis* 60: 357–373.

Persons, J.B. (1989) *Cognitive Therapy in Practice: A Case Formulation Approach*. New York: W.W. Norton.

Racker, H. (1957) The meanings and uses of countertransference. *Psychoanalytic Quarterly* 26: 303–357.

—— (1968) *Transference and Countertransference*. London: Hogarth Press.

Rayner, E. (1991) *The Independent Mind in British Psychoanalysis*. London: Free Association Books.

Regina, P. (1997) Memory: Brain systems that link past, present and future. *International Journal of Psycho-Analysis* 78: 1223–1234.

Renik, O. (1993) Analytic interaction: conceptualizing technique in light of the analyst's irreducible subjectivity. *Psychoanalytic Quarterly* 62: 553–571.

Richards, A.K. (1997) The relevance of frequency of sessions to the creation of an analytic experience. *Journal of the American Psychoanalytic Association* 45: 1241–1251.

Rosenfeld, H. (1987) *Impasse and Interpretation*. London: Tavistock Publications.

Roughton, R.E. (1993) Useful aspects of acting out: repetition, enactment, and actualization. *Journal of the American Psychoanalytic Association* 41: 443–472.

Ruderman, E., Shane, E. and Shane, M. (eds) (2000) On touch in the psychoanalytic situation. *Psychoanalytic Inquiry* 20(1).

Sandler, J. (1976) Countertransference and role-responsiveness. *International Review of Psycho-Analysis* 3: 43–47.

—— (1993) On communication from patient to analyst: not everything is projective identification. *International Journal of Psycho-Analysis* 74: 1097–1107.

Searles, H.F. (1959) The effort to drive the other person crazy: an element in the aetiology and psychotherapy of schizophrenia. *British Journal of Medical Psychology* 32: 1–18.

—— (1965) *Collected Papers on Schizophrenia and Related Subjects*. London: Hogarth Press.

—— (1975) The patient as therapist to his analyst, in P.L. Giovacchini (ed.), *Tactics and Techniques in Psychoanalytic Therapy, Vol. 11*. New York: Jason Aronson.

Sinason, V. (ed.) (1994) *Treating Survivors of Satanist Abuse*. London: Routledge.

—— (ed.) (1998) *Memory in Dispute*. London: Karnac.

Snyder, S. (1993) Meeting of the Psychoanalytic Association of New York. *Psychoanalytic Quarterly* 62: 704.

Sterba, R. (1934) The fate of the ego in analytic therapy. *International Journal of Psycho-Analysis* 15: 117–26.

Winnicott, D.W. (1941) The observation of infants in a set situation. *International Journal of Psycho-Analysis* 22: 229–249.

—— (1954a) Withdrawal and regression, in D.W. Winnicott (1958) *Collected Papers: Through Paediatrics to Psycho-Analysis*. London: Tavistock Publications, pp. 255–261.

—— (1954b) Metapsychological and clinical aspects of regression within the psycho-analytical set-up, in D.W. Winnicott (1958) *Collected Papers: Through Paediatrics to Psycho-Analysis*. London: Tavistock Publications, pp. 278–294.

—— (1955) Metapsychological and clinical aspects of regression within the psycho-analytical set-up. *International Journal of Psycho-Analysis* 36: 16–26.

—— (1956) On transference. *International Journal of Psycho-Analysis* 37: 386–388.

—— (1958) *Collected Papers: Through Paediatrics to Psycho-Analysis*. London: Tavistock Publications.

—— (1962) Ego integration in child development, in D.W. Winnicott (1965) *The Maturational Process and the Facilitating Environment*. London: Hogarth Press, pp. 56–63.

—— (1963a) Psychiatric disorder in terms of infantile maturational processes, in D.W. Winnicott (1965) *The Maturational Processes and the Facilitating Environment*. London: Hogarth Press, pp. 230–241.

—— (1963b) Dependence in infant care, in child care, and in the psycho-analytic setting. *International Journal of Psycho-Analysis* 44: 339–344.

—— (1965a) A clinical study of the effect of a failure of the average expectable environment on a child's mental functioning. *International Journal of Psycho-Analysis* 46: 81–87.

—— (1965b) *The Maturational Processes and the Facilitating Environment.* London: Hogarth Press.

—— (1967) Mirror-role of mother and family in child development, in P. Lomas (ed.), *The Predicament of the Family.* London: Hogarth Press.

—— (1971a) *Therapeutic Consultations in Child Psychiatry.* London: Hogarth Press.

—— (1971b) *Playing and Reality.* London: Tavistock Publications.

—— (1974) Fear of breakdown. *International Review of Psycho-Analysis* 1: 103–107.

—— (1988) *Human Nature.* London: Free Association Books.

Name index

Alexander, F. 85
Aron, Lewis 5*n*, 87*n*

Balint, Michael 86, 90, 129
Beck, J. 123*n*
Bion, Wilfred R. 65–6, 100, 115*n*,
  123, 125, 136–7, 138–9
Blum, Harold P. 98*n*
Boesky, D. 87*n*
Bollas, Christopher 122
Breckenridge, K. 90, 91
Breuer, J. 3
Britton, Ronald 100*n*
Bromberg, Philip 98*n*

Chused, Judith 17–18, 72*n*

Eissler, K. R. 131*n*
Emmy von N., Frau 3

Fiscalini, John 9*n*
Fosshage, J. L. 89
Fox, R. P. 87*n*
Freud, Sigmund 2–3, 9, 41*n*, 103

Greenberg, Jay 101

Heimann, Paula 43–4, 43*n*, 92
Hobson, R. F. 100*n*
Hoffer, A. 87*n*

Katz, G. A. 87*n*
Keller, Helen 116–17
Kernberg, Otto 14
Kirsner, D. 14*n*
Klein, Melanie 32, 88*n*, 104*n*

Kohon, G. 86*n*

Ladan, A. 31*n*
Langs, Robert J. 9*n*, 18*n*, 22, 28–9, 49
Levenson, E. A. 17*n*
Lewis, E. 72
Little, Margaret 71, 86, 129

Marrone, M. 100*n*
Meares, R. A. 100*n*
Meissner, W. W. 87*n*
Mitchell, Stephen 2*n*

Ogden, T. 137

Persons, J. B. 123*n*

Racker, H. 35, 137
Raphling, David 17–18
Rayner, E. 34*n*
Regina, P. 124*n*
Renik, Owen 72*n*
Richards, Arlene K. 98*n*
Rock, M. H. 43
Rosenfeld, H. 12
Roughton, R. E. 87

Sandler, Joseph 32, 72, 137, 138
Searles, Harold F. 13, 22
Snyder, Steven 98*n*
Sterba, R. 25
Sullivan, Annie 116–17

Winnicott, Donald W. 7–8, 9, 13–14,
  28*n*, 33, 37, 71, 83, 85, 86, 89, 90,
  96–7, 104, 105, 112, 123, 129,
  130*n*, 137, 138

Subject index

abandonment, coping with summer break, clinical example 60–1

abstracting, need to abstract essential theme from detail, clinical example 52–3

aggressor, identification with 15

analyst: analyst–patient relationship, and mother–infant relationship 112–13; internal dialogue 24–7; need to promote healthy relating 10

analytic curiosity 100

analytic space: encouraging revelation of psychotic areas 11–13; environmental factors 14, 96–7, 104–5; Freud's discovery 2–3; and impingement, avoidance of 100–9; opening up, clinical example 51–2; playing and being 105–6; problem of Freud's fundamental rule 2–3; theoretical views inform attitude to 104–5, *see also* impingement

anger, patient able to give expression to after sessions rearranged 66–70

autonomy: supervisee's fostering of internal supervision 43–57, *see also* internal supervision

avoidance 101*n*; misuse of interpretation 4

blank screen 103–4

boundary issues, keeping to and breaking rules 28–32

cancellation (analyst's): explaining reasons for, clinical example 63–4; feeling of insecurity following, clinical example 53–4

certainty: as imprisonment 16, *see also* sureness

clinical examples: analysis without interpretation 124–5; analyst's re-enactment, success by failing 72–85; analytic space 101–4, 106–9; being helpful, patient's reading of analyst's motivation 61–2, 66–70; boundary issues, accepting gifts 29–32; break, dealing with feelings of abandonment 60–1; cancellation, explaining reasons for 63–4; communicating experience, detailed clinical presentation 34–42; confidentiality, therapeutic value 11–12; deflecting from difficult matter 49–50; discomfort of silence 25–6; displacement, result of analyst's defensiveness 48–9; finding a bridge to understand the unknown 117–22; insecurity, following cancellation of session 53–4; interpretation as threat 56; intrusion 10; mothering, unexpected reaction to concept of 114–15; need to abstract essential theme from detail 52–3; negative transference, development of deflected 48–9; not-knowing

stance to encourage reflection
54–6; Oedipal triumph, boundary
issue 29–30; perception, analyst's
and patient's 51–2; physical
contact, appropriateness of 85–95,
129–39; punctuality, analyst's
attempt to make good lateness
62–3; reassurance, alternative to
60–1; self-proving 5–6; therapist
mistakenly introducing material
50–1; unconscious criticism of
patient 25–7; violence, phantasy
and reality 49–50
communication: deaf, blind and
mute student 116–17; derivative
communication, boundary issue
29; interpretation as unconscious
communication 9; silence as
97n
compliance: and false-self 97–8;
inappropriate interpretations 7, 14;
problem of in psychoanalytic
training 1–16
confidentiality, as therapeutic, clinical
example 11–12
confrontation, needs of patients 8
containment, failure to deal with
phantasy of violence 49–50
contrast, unconscious criticism by
patient 22, 27
correction, need for analyst to be
open to 4
countertransference: before and after
qualification 46; consideration of
in light of mistakes 32; fear of the
contained, clinical example 136–7;
indirect countertransference 35,
137; personal and diagnostic 32,
see also transference

denial, misuse of interpretation 4
depressive position, mis-
interpretation of compliance 13
derivative communication, Langs on
29
displacement: clinical example 49;
misuse of interpretation 4;
unconscious criticism by patient
22, 27

dogmatism 14n; as persecutory 19;
and tentativeness 19–21, see also
sureness

ego: analyst's observing ego and
participating ego 25; weakened by
interpretations 13
enactment: analyst's re-enactment,
clinical example 71–85;
co-creation of transference 98n
environmental factors, effects of
impinging environment 14, 96–7,
104–5
envy 104; of the good breast 104n
experience, and theory, understanding
the unknown 112–14, 122–3
exploration, and interpretations 18

failing: success by failing, clinical
example 72–85; Winnicott on 33,
71, 89, 138
false-self, and compliance 15, 97–8
firmness see sureness
Fort...Da game 41n
free association, Freud's insistence
upon 3
free-floating responsiveness 72
fundamental rule (Freud's), and
analytic space 2–3

good experience, distress in midst of
121

helping, hazards in being helpful
58–70
hesitation, period of important to
infant 7

identification, trial identification 5
impasse, hazards in being helpful
59
impingement 96–109; and analytic
space 100–4; definition 96n; and
the environment 14, 96–7, 104–5;
objects as meaningful or as
impingement 7, see also analytic
space
implicit memory 124n
independence see autonomy

indirect countertransference 35, 137
infants: impingement 96–7; period
    of hesitation 7; and regression 7
insecurity, feeling of insecurity
    following cancellation of session
    53–4
insight 18
intellectualizing: clinical example 56,
    see also theory
internal supervision: internal dialogue
    as 24–5; supervisee's fostering of
    autonomy 46–7
interpersonal dimensions, analytic
    interaction 5
interpretations: co-creation of
    transference 98n; danger of
    compliance 14; error as intrinsic
    aspect of analytic situation 18;
    importance of play 7–8, 14;
    inappropriate use of as
    impingement 98–9; as indication
    of limit of understanding 28n;
    knowing and not-knowing 27–8;
    need to maintain analytic space
    101, 105–9; as unconscious
    communications 9
intolerable situation, danger of
    therapist trying to relieve tension
    65–6
introjective reference, unconscious
    criticism by patient 23, 27
intrusion: avoiding in analytic
    relationship 10; importance of
    period of hesitation 7–8; resistance
    to deep interpretation 5

knowledge: and caution of using
    knowledge 15; illusion of 117, see
    also not-knowing

masturbation, therapist's
    embarrassment, failure to open up
    analytic space 51–2
memory 124
mind of ones own, problem in
    analytic training 2
mirroring: mother's face as mirror 37;
    unconscious criticism by patient
    23

mistakes 17–33; admitting to or not
    32–3; avoiding, detailed clinical
    presentation 34–42; examining
    countertransference 32; as part of
    analytic process or not 33; success
    in failure 71–85
mother–infant relationship: and
    analyst–patient relationship
    112–13; mother's face as mirror
    37; mother's role in accepting
    projections 65–6, 138; playing
    105; seduction 7
mothering, unexpected reaction
    to concept, clinical example
    114–15

nameless dread, as result of
    projections not accepted 66, 70,
    138
needs, firmness and limits 8–9
negative view of patients 99
neutrality 101
not-knowing: interpretations 27–8;
    stance of to encourage reflection,
    clinical example 54–6; value of
    123–5

objective realities, and transference
    101, 103
objects, infants discern as meaningful
    or as an impingement 7
Oedipus complex, boundary issue,
    clinical example 29–30
other: otherness of 116–17; as
    unknown 114–15

pathologizing, students who disagree
    15
patients: unconscious criticism by
    21–7; unconscious supervision by
    49
penetrative, interpretations as 5
persecutory anxiety, and persecution
    10, 12
phantasy, difficulty of dealing with
    potential violence, clinical example
    50–1
physical contact, clinical example
    86–95

play: infant finding the mother 105; understanding clinical material 18*n*; use of interpretations 7–8

Playing and Reality (Winnicott) 14, 105

pressure: Freud's fundamental rule as impugning analytic space 2–3; pressure of authority 15

projection: misuse of interpretation 4; mother's role in detoxifying 65–6

projective identification 88*n*; evoking unbearable state in analyst 137; experience of not being able to see, clinical example 118; feelings of helplessness, clinical example 135; misuse of interpretation 4; mother's failure to tolerate infant's projections 65–6, 138

projective-identification-rejecting-object 136–7

psychotic areas in patient, approaches to 11–13

punctuality, therapist late for session, clinical examples 52–3, 62–3

reassurance, danger of and alternative to 60–1

regression: deep regression and appropriateness of physical contact 86; and infancy 7

rejection, idea of mistakenly introduced, clinical example 50–1

resistance: healthy resistance 19; interpretation of to explain disagreement 3

reversal, misuse of interpretation 4

role-responsiveness 72, 137

security, feeling of insecurity following cancellation of session 53–4

seduction, of infants 7

separation anxiety, mis-interpretation of 6

Shadow of the Object, The, (Bollas) 122

silence, as communication 97*n*

space *see* analytic space

spatula, infants' reaction to 7–8

splitting, misuse of interpretation 4

squiggle game 8

style 18–19

suffering, uniqueness of other's suffering 116

supervision: autonomy, fostering use of internal supervision 43–57; internal dialogue as internal supervision 24–5; problems in supervisory triad 44–6

sureness: danger of self-proving, clinical example 5–7; inappropriate sureness leading to deflection of issue, clinical example 54–6; inappropriate tentativeness, clinical example 53–4; making correction difficult 20; misuse of interpretations 3–4; need for analyst to be open to correction 4; and problem of compliance 2, 14–15; and tentativeness 19–21

technique: errors as intrinsic aspect of analytic situation 17–18; Freud's development of 2–3

tension, attempt to relieve experienced as deflecting the unmanageable 65–6

tentativeness: and sureness 19–21; value of stance of not-knowing, clinical example 54–6

theory: aid to understanding the unknown 112–14; different attitudes to analytic space 104–5; need for balance, understanding unique individual 122–3

timelessness of the unconscious, misuse of interpretation 4

training, pressure in analysis to comply 1–16

transference: analyst trying to be helpful, clinical example 62–3; analyst's attempt to relieve tension 66; co-creation of 98*n*; interpretations of 4, 8, 47; negative transference, patient deflected from developing 49, 53; and objective realities 101, 103, *see also* countertransference

transference–countertransference
relationship 9*n*
trauma, feeling in present earlier
trauma 137
trial identification 5, 20–1, 42;
encouraging student's use of 47–9;
internal dialogue 25

unconscious supervision by patient
21–7, 55; Langs on 22, 49
unknown 110–25; getting to know the
other, clinical examples 116–22;

relating to the unfamiliar 110–12;
theory, contribution and limitation
of 112–14, 122–3; uniqueness of
the other 114–16; value of not-
knowing 123–5
unmanageable feelings, physical
contact used to avoid confronting,
clinical example 86–95
unthinkable anxieties 130*n*
unthought known 122

working alliance, enabling 18–19